A Cancer Prevention Guide for the Human Race

Robert A. Wascher, MD, FACS

This book is to be used for informational purposes only, and it is not intended to substitute for the advice or recommendations of your personal physician.

All readers should seek the advice of their physician <u>before</u> making any changes in their medications, diet, or level of physcial activity.

First published by Dog Ear Publishing
4010 W. 86th Street, Ste H
Indianapolis, IN 46268
www.dogearpublishing.net

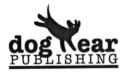

ISBN: 978-160844-691-9

This book is printed on acid-free paper.

Printed in the United States of America

DEDICATION

I dedicate this book to the thousands of patients who, over the past 25 years, I have been privileged to care for. Their valiant and determined battles against cancer have always left me with a sense of awe and respect at the power and beauty and strength of the human spirit. The dignity and grace with which they have fought to conquer their cancers have also inspired to me to always remember what is really important in life (and what is not important).

I also dedicate this book to my beloved Dominique, and to our cherished and precious Alexis and Aaron. Thank you for bringing the joy, the laughter, the colors, the sounds, the richness, and all of the memories into my life that have so completely transformed me over the past 15 years. Most of all, thank you for your love and your steadfast support, day after day. You have made my life complete.

TABLE OF CONTENTS

Part I

A Comprehensive Guide to Cancer Biology

& Cancer Prevention

Part II

Expanded Clinical Cancer Section

Part III

PART I

A COMPREHENSIVE GUIDE TO CANCER

BIOLOGY & CANCER PREVENTION

CHAPTER 1

INTRODUCTION

Few, if any, diseases evoke a greater sense of dread than cancer. Patients newly diagnosed with cancer often react with a combination of fear and disbelief, and with a powerful and sudden realization that nothing is promised to any of us beyond the current moment.

Over the past 30 years, significant progress has been made in treating cancer. Based upon recent cancer survival statistics, an unprecedented 65 percent of all patients newly diagnosed with cancer are likely to be alive and clinically cancer-free 5 years later (for most types of cancer, being free of residual or recurrent cancer for 5 years is considered to be the clinical equivalent of a cure). However, the emotional, physical, and financial costs of cancer remain very high even for long-term cancer survivors, and for their loved ones. While an increasing number of cancer patients are becoming long-term survivors, cancer continues to take a heavy toll on the lives of both the young and the old throughout the world.

Despite continuing advances in cancer treatment, cancer is still a very frequent cause of death. For the nearly 600,000 patients in the United States, alone, who died of cancer in 2009, and for whom cure was therefore not possible, only cancer *prevention* could have potentially prevented some of these premature deaths. While not every case of cancer can be prevented (or cured), recent clinical research findings suggest that, conservatively, 40 to 65 percent of all cases of cancer, including some of the deadliest forms of cancer, can be prevented with prudent and relatively moderate lifestyle and diet changes. Therefore, when it comes to the issue of cancer prevention, the old adage about an ounce of prevention being worth a pound of cure should probably be revised to, "An *ounce* of cancer prevention is worth a *ton* of cancer cure."

Before I begin my comprehensive discussion of evidence-based cancer prevention lifestyle and diet strategies, I must first offer a few words of caution. We live in a truly wondrous age where information about almost any subject can be effortlessly and instantaneously acquired from a variety of sources. Unfortunately, the sheer volume and complexity of the health-related information at hand can challenge even the most knowledgeable among us when trying to separate valid information from useless (and sometimes dangerous) anecdotes, over-simplifications, and transient fads. The unfortunate reality is that much, if not most, of the health-related information that is presented in the popular media, including the Internet, is based primarily upon anecdotal evidence, badly performed science, junk science, no science at all, or "cherry-picked" science.

One must always remember that the Worldwide Web, which has revolutionized the global dissemination of information, remains a completely unfiltered source of health information. Therefore, consumers of health information have to be especially cautious when evaluating the plethora of claims and recommendations available on the Internet, and from other public sources of information. (As one should, indeed, not judge a book by its cover, so it is that one should also not judge the accuracy of the content of a website by how "professional" the site appears to be.)

One should also not judge the validity of health-related theories and claims made by self-anointed "experts" based solely upon the number of degrees that appear behind their names. Similarly, the use of celebrity spokespersons to advocate for (or against) particular diets or treatments is a common practice, and one that is rife with oversimplification, misrepresentation, and outright fraud. To put it rather bluntly, there is an enormous volume of bad health-related information to be found wherever one looks, including on the Internet, on television, and in many popular magazines and books.

As just one example, take the bestselling book by an author who describes herself as an "independent research scientist" (actually, it appears that she obtained a Ph.D. degree in Zoology in 1958, and has had no subsequent clinical research affiliations with any major university or medical center during the past 30 years). In her book, which currently enjoys the lofty Amazon.com sales rank of #9,183, she makes the jaw-dropping claim that modern science has somehow failed to discover, as she has, that *all cancers are actually caused by a single human parasite,* and that, therefore, all cancers can be cured by eradicating this parasite with her proprietary diet plan and herbal supplements!

Other books, tabloid articles, television infomercials, and websites often make equally bizarre or far-fetched claims about cancer-preventing or cancer-curing diets, vitamins, dietary supplements, homeopathic remedies, body cavity cleansings, medical contraptions, and numerous other unproven nostrums. Many of these unproven "alternative" remedies are also energetically endorsed by vivacious celebrities, or by earnest-looking people with advanced degrees, thereby adding a veneer of respectability to these sales pitches (although the spokespersons for these remedies, even when they have advanced degrees, almost always lack any direct background in mainstream laboratory or clinical cancer research).

In view of the highly confusing health information landscape out there, this book has been written with the goal of offering health-conscious readers a comprehensive, objective, research-based review of lifestyle and dietary strategies known to reduce the risk of developing the types of cancer that, together, cause the great majority of all cancer-associated deaths.

It should always be remembered that, despite the many ludicrous promises that have been made to miraculously prevent or cure virtually every case of cancer, *there are no magical formulas* that, at the present time, will prevent or cure 100 percent of all cancers. Fortunately, however, there is a growing body of high-level clinical research that offers all of us a rational and evidence-based approach to minimizing our risk of developing cancer.

One must be cautious when interpreting clinical research findings, however. For example, based upon seemingly compelling research findings, there is a huge appetite for vitamin supplements in the United States, and in other countries around the world. Millions of people take vitamins and dietary supplements in the hope that these supplements will ward off disease, including cancer, and improve both their health and their lifespan. However, the bulk of the enthusiastic "scientific claims" made for many vitamins and dietary supplements are based primarily upon very low-powered public health research studies.

In addition to low-powered and bias-prone survey-based public health research studies, much of the published cancer prevention research data suggesting a positive role for vitamins, dietary supplements, or special diets, has been based upon other relatively low-powered research methods, including studies of human cancer cells growing in culture dishes, and the implantation of human tumors into laboratory mice that are genetically engineered to have a faulty immune system (an important consideration, as we know that our immune system plays a very important role in cancer prevention, as well as in the body's response to many cancer treatments). Unfortunately, there have been, literally, hundreds of potentially promising treatments identified by these types of laboratory research studies that have subsequently gone on to be proven worthless when studied in humans (worse yet, some of these therapies have actually proven to be toxic to humans). However, because prospective, randomized, placebo-controlled clinical studies are so expensive and time-consuming to perform, these less rigorous methods of cancer prevention research still have an important role to play in our search for more effective methods of preventing and treating cancer. In view of their serious limitations, however, these inexpensive and rapid methods of research are best utilized to screen potentially promising cancer prevention and treatment approaches that are worthy of further evaluation using very expensive and time-consuming prospective, randomized human clinical studies. Over the past 10 years, an increasing number of large-scale prospective, randomized, placebo-controlled cancer prevention trials have been performed, and these high-level research studies have increasingly called into question the clinical value of many of the vitamins and other dietary supplements that previously were thought to have a potential role in preventing cancer. (Ironically, some of the most frequently touted "cancer prevention" vitamins and dietary supplements have actually been shown, recently, to *increase* health risks, including the risk of some of the very same cancers that they were supposed to prevent!)

In my view, it is important to critically evaluate the findings of clinical research studies that are based upon relatively weak methodologies, and to avoid accepting the results of such studies at face value. As just one of many examples of how the favorable findings of low-level clinical research studies can be reversed by high-quality prospective clinical research trials, the uniformly disappointing results of several recent large prospective clinical trials looking at the use of certain antioxidant vitamins (and other dietary antioxidant supplements) to prevent both cancer and cardiovascular disease have caused many public health experts to stop recommending these supplements. Although prior research on the biochemical effects of these antioxidant nutrients (using human cancer cells grown in a culture dish, or human tumors implanted into mice with compromised immune systems) had suggested that these dietary agents might be useful in preventing cancer in humans, several recent large-scale randomized, placebo-controlled, blinded, prospective human research trials have revealed *no detectable cancer prevention benefit associated with selenium, Vitamin E, Vitamin C, or Vitamin A (and other members of the Vitamin A family)*. Moreover, as I will discuss later in this book, several of these very large prospective clinical trials have actually uncovered an *increased risk of cancer*, and even death, among large numbers of study volunteers who were randomized to take some of these antioxidant vitamins.

Fortunately, despite the disappointing results of recent large-scale prospective human cancer prevention trials, there is still tremendous potential for health-conscious people to drastically reduce their lifetime risk of developing cancer, and to minimize their overall risk of dying from cancer. In this book, which is written for readers without a formal medical or scientific background, you will find a treasure trove of valuable cancer biology and cancer prevention information. In every case, the information provided in this book is derived from extensive laboratory and clinical research data that has been published in high-quality peer-reviewed medical textbooks and journals. This book is the result of an exhaustive review of, literally, hundreds of such research studies, conducted by thousands of the world's most prominent experts in cancer biology and cancer prevention.

Whenever possible, I have preferentially cited the findings of prospective, randomized, placebo-controlled clinical research studies, which remain the "gold standard" method of performing clinical research, and which are the only source of so-called "Level 1" clinical evidence. In those cases where no "Level 1" clinical research evidence is available, I have also included studies based upon less rigorous forms of research, while also taking care to point out the limitations of many of these lower-powered studies. This honest, evidence-based approach to cancer prevention is the standard by which all other lifestyle- and diet-based disease prevention books must be measured (and precious few of them live up to this standard, unfortunately). This scientific, evidence-based approach to cancer prevention, based upon an exhaustive review of the available clinical and scientific research on cancer prevention, makes this book an extreme rarity among the tiny number of comprehensive cancer prevention books that have been published for the lay public over the past 50 years.

Today, and for the foreseeable future, cancer prevention remains a far more effective public health strategy than treating cancers once they have already developed. Consequently, the prime objective of this book is to arm health-conscious readers with a concise, comprehensive, and highly readable summary of the latest evidence-based research data available on preventing the most common types of cancer that, together, account for the majority of all cancer deaths in the United States, and throughout much of the world as well.

CHAPTER 2

AN OVERVIEW OF CANCER

Cancer Epidemiology

Before discussing evidence-based strategies for cancer prevention, let us first consider the scope of cancer as a public health problem. Based upon statistics compiled by the American Cancer Society, 1 of every 2 men, and 1 of every 3 women, in the United States will be diagnosed with cancer during their lifetime. In 2010, an estimated 1.5 million Americans will be diagnosed with cancer. Nearly 600,000 Americans will also die of cancer in 2010, accounting for one 1 out of every 4 deaths in the United States. According to the American Cancer Society, there are also more than 11 million cancer survivors currently living in the United States, many of whom are at increased risk of developing new or recurrent cancers [1].

As a testament to the relatively greater success that has been achieved in reducing the death rate from cardiovascular disease, cancer has already replaced cardiovascular disease as the #1 killer of Americans under the age of 85, according to recent American Cancer Society statistics [2]. Cancer is also projected to soon become the #1 cause of death world-wide, as well. In December of 2008, the International Agency for Research on Cancer, which is part of the United Nations World Health Organization, forecasted that cancer is expected to overtake cardiovascular disease and infectious diseases to become *the most common cause of death throughout the world in 2010.*

Recently, some modest progress has been made in turning back the historically rising incidence of cancer in the United States, and in decreasing cancer-associated death rates. A recently published update of cancer statistics, collected between 1975 and 2005, and jointly published by the American Cancer Society, the National Cancer Institute, and the Centers for Disease Control, provides important insights into the tremendous potential of cancer prevention and cancer screening strategies to reduce cancer-associated deaths in our society [3]. This comprehensive new cancer incidence and mortality update reveals that, *for the first time* ever, a modest but significant *decrease* in the incidence of new cancers was noted in the United States between 2002 and 2005. During this period, the annual number of new cancer cases declined by just under 1 percent per year, suggesting that, finally, we are beginning to see improved compliance with established cancer prevention and cancer screening guidelines. During the same 3-year period, the overall cancer-associated death rate also decreased by almost 2 percent per year. This modest but historic decline in cancer incidence, as well as the continuing downward trend in cancer deaths, can be attributed primarily to the incremental but sustained improvements in cancer prevention, cancer screening, and cancer treatment that have been achieved over the past 15 to 20 years.

But not all of the news contained in this landmark cancer epidemiology report was good news, unfortunately. For, although cancer-associated death rates for 10 of the 15 most common types of cancer modestly declined between 2002 and 2005, cancer death rates actually *increased* for cancers of the esophagus, bladder, pancreas, and liver.

Even among some types of cancer for which the overall death rates have been declining, there is still some unfavorable news to be found. For example, the overall death rate due to lung cancer has been slowly declining for more than a decade now in the United States. However, when you look more carefully at the statistics for the #1 cancer killer throughout most of the world (including the United States), the picture becomes a bit more complicated. The death rate due to lung cancer in the United States has indeed been gradually declining since the early 1990s, *but only for men* (following many years of declining smoking rates among men). During this same period, however, smoking rates among women were rising, and so the incidence of lung cancer-related deaths among women have, not surprisingly, continued to increase, even as lung cancer deaths have fallen among men.

Also, there are significant regional differences in cancer incidence and cancer-associated death trends in the United States. California stands out as the undisputed pioneer in legislating restrictions against smoking in public places, and in funding comprehensive anti-smoking public education programs. (In 1995, California enacted the first statewide ordinance outlawing smoking in public places.) Once again, taking lung cancer as an example, we see that lung cancer death rates *declined* by almost 3 percent per year in California between

1996 and 2005, which is about *twice* the rate of decline that was observed among most Midwestern and Southern states during the same period. Thus, these statistics clearly demonstrate that lifestyle modifications can have a *dramatic* impact upon the incidence of certain cancers, and upon the death rates associated with these same cancers.

These data, and data from numerous other similar cancer research studies, show that, without a doubt, we need to do more to prevent those cases of cancer that can be prevented (and to diagnose, at the earliest possible stage, those cancer cases that could not be prevented).

As our population in the United States, and in other parts of the world, becomes both older and more diverse, the incidence of cancer is expected to rise even further over the next two decades. A recent study evaluated demographic trends, as well as data from a large national cancer database, to estimate future trends in cancer incidence within the United States. Based upon this data, by 2030 there will be an estimated 365 million people living in the United States, including 72 million adults aged 65 years or older. Additionally, an estimated 157 million Americans are predicted to be members of minority ethnic groups. Based upon data that consistently shows a higher cancer incidence among the elderly and among members of ethnic minority groups, the authors of this epidemiological study estimate that, between 2010 and 2030, the total incidence of cancer will *increase by a whopping 45 percent* (from 1.5 million forecasted new cancer cases in 2010, to a projected 2.3 million new cases in 2030). Because the risk of developing cancer significantly increases with advancing age, the number of new cancer cases among elderly Americans, specifically, is predicted to *increase by a stunning 67 percent* between 2010 and 2030. Moreover, due to the increasing number of people from ethnic minority backgrounds in the United States, and the increasing average age of minority populations (as with the population as a whole), the number of cancer cases among the non-Caucasian population in the United States is projected to *increase by an astonishing 99 percent* between 2010 and 2030, compared with a predicted 31 percent increase in cancer cases within the Caucasian population. These alarming projections are a stark reminder that we must do much more to modify our lifestyles and diets in order to eliminate as many preventable cases of cancer as is possible [4].

Based upon current cancer incidence trends, approximately 40 percent of Americans will be diagnosed with cancer during their lifetimes [5]. In fact, cancer has become such a common illness that more than half of us will be personally touched by this disease during the course of our lives, either by becoming cancer patients ourselves, or through our close relationships with others who have become cancer patients. Therefore, the time for all of us to change from a "cancer-prone" lifestyle to a "cancer-prevention" lifestyle and diet is right now!

Cancer Biology

The term "cancer" is actually an umbrella diagnosis that includes an estimated 150 separate and distinct diseases, all of which share some important common biological features. Generally speaking, cancers are diseases that are characterized by the presence of abnormal cells that have become transformed, or "immortalized," allowing these mutated cells to divide and reproduce indefinitely (unlike normal cells that naturally die after a predetermined number of cell divisions). Because of these abnormal biological traits, cancer cells can continue to divide until they form a mass, or tumor. But several other critical biological traits must also be acquired by cancer cells before they are capable of causing significant harm to their host. Because tumors require increasing amounts of oxygen and other nutrients as they enlarge, most cancerous tumors also secrete proteins that stimulate the development and growth of new blood vessels from the tumor's periphery. (A tiny one centimeter tumor, barely one-third of an inch around, already contains approximately one billion malignant cells!) However, most people who die from cancer do not die due to the presence of a single tumor, however large. Rather, the most important clinical feature of cancer cells is that, unlike normal cells in our bodies, cancer cells are able to invade and spread throughout the body, and to colonize vital organs with their malignant progeny, until their host eventually becomes overwhelmed. Thus, in order to cause the "clinical disease" of cancer, malignant cells from the primary tumor must first invade surrounding normal tissues, and then gain access to the blood vessels and lymphatic channels that can then transport them to distant sites throughout the body. Once viable cancer cells have arrived at their far-flung destinations, these malignant cells must then egress from their vascular super-highways and then, once again, invade through surrounding normal tissues and organs, and then go on to develop metastatic tumors. Above all, it is this metastatic capability of cancer cells that causes the vast majority of all cancer-associated deaths.

Despite the fact that cancer is so commonly diagnosed, the odds *against* individual cancer cells surviving and successfully metastasizing are actually

amazingly high. As potential cancer cells acquire successively more gene mutations, the vast majority of them will undergo a form of suicidal cell death,
known as apoptosis, before they can spread, due to the accumulation of lethal
mutations. Moreover, additional dangers lurk everywhere within our bodies
for aspiring cancer cells that manage to avoid these lethal internal genetic
mutations. The white blood cells and antibodies of our immune system are
constantly on the prowl for aberrant, mutated cells, and destroy most of these
abnormal cells almost immediately. The tiny fraction of cancer cells that successfully evade the immune system's surveillance and onslaught are the malignant cells that are most likely to, ultimately, go on to produce the clinical
syndromes that we associate with cancer.

The recent pace of medical and scientific discovery has reached a previously
unimaginable level. Following the unraveling of the human genetic code, or
human genome, in 2003, our progress in understanding the genetic and biochemical machinery of both normal and cancerous cells has accelerated enormously. Increasingly, it has become apparent that most cancer cells arise from
normal precursor cells as a result of critical mutations within small numbers of
very specific genes. The majority of these mutations occur within the estimated 5 percent of our genes that directly regulate the critical processes of
DNA repair, cell division, and cell death within every one of the 50 to 75 tril-
lion cells in our bodies. Mutations in these critical regulatory genes arise from
a variety of mechanisms, and result in the loss of DNA integrity in affected
cells. When characteristic mutations occur in highly specific genes, the resulting "transformed" cells may then begin to acquire the biological traits that
allow them to cause the clinical disease known as cancer. When one consid-
ers that an estimated 10,000 DNA-damaging biological events occur in *every*
cell of our body each and every day, one begins to understand the remarkable
efficiency and accuracy of the DNA repair mechanisms in the trillions of cells
throughout our body. When these complex surveillance and repair systems
fail in critically mutated cells within our bodies, however, the result is, very
often, a new cancer.

Finally, while the vast majority of new cancers appear to arise from a single
mutated "parent" cell in our bodies, some cancer-producing DNA mutations
can actually be inherited from our parents and, in turn, can also be passed
down to our sons and daughters. Currently, it is estimated that 85 to 90 percent of all cases of cancer arise sporadically. That is to say, a series of sporadic
(random) and sequential genetic mutational events accumulate within a *single*
cell, and these events, in turn, transform that afflicted cell into a cancer cell.

In contrast to sporadic cancers, however, somewhere between 10 and 15 percent of cancers are currently known to arise not from acquired mutations in the DNA of a single cell, but rather due to inherited genetic mutations that are present in the DNA of *every cell in the body*.

In all cases of cancer, however, mutations in genes that critically regulate cell reproduction, DNA repair, and cell death cause a transformation of previously normal cells to occur. These transformed cells, with their disabled DNA repair systems, then go on to acquire additional mutations in other critical genes as well, until, ultimately, one or more of these cells become cancer cells. Indeed, as I often say when I am lecturing to medical students and residents, "All cancer is genetic."

Current Approaches to Cancer Treatment

Surgery, Chemotherapy & Molecularly-Targeted Therapies

For the vast majority of cancers that form solid tumors, surgical resection remains the single most effective available treatment, particularly for early-stage cancers. Adjuvant, or supplementary, cancer therapies are also often used in a multidisciplinary approach to cancer treatment, and include chemotherapy, radiation therapy and, sometimes, hormonal therapy. While none of these adjuvant therapies are as effective as the surgical removal of all detectable traces of tumor, they are nonetheless additive to the beneficial effects of surgery in reducing the risk of cancer recurrence, and death due to cancer.

Since the dawn of the chemotherapy era, in the 1940s, most chemotherapy drugs have relied upon their differential toxic effects with respect to cancer cells and normal cells. Even today, the standard "cytotoxic" chemotherapy drugs commonly in use are toxic to virtually all of the body's cells, as these drugs target the same essential biological pathways that are necessary for the survival of both cancer cells and normal cells. In general, these drugs preferentially target critical biochemical pathways that are required for cell growth and reproduction. However, fortunately, because these biochemical pathways are far more active in rapidly dividing cancer cells (i.e., compared to most normal cells), the toxic effects of these chemotherapy drugs are more pronounced against cancer cells. (The toxicity of cancer chemotherapies towards rapidly dividing normal cells accounts for most of chemotherapy's unpleasant side-effects, including nausea, vomiting, diarrhea, sores of the mouth and GI tract, loss of appetite, weight loss, and hair loss. Other clinically important toxicities of standard chemotherapy drugs include infertility, changes in taste, skin rashes, discoloration of the fingernails and toenails, sensory disturbances, heart failure, kidney failure, and potentially serious liver abnormalities.)

Recently, we have entered a new era in adjuvant cancer therapy, sometimes referred to as the Molecular Era. As our understanding of the genetic and biochemical machinery of both normal cells and cancer cells has continued to expand, we are discovering an increasing number of genetic and biochemical abnormalities that are, in fact, relatively specific to the biology of cancer cells. Based upon this newfound and still-expanding frontier of knowledge, we are increasingly able to exploit these genetic and biochemical cancer cell derangements by designing "molecularly-targeted" therapies. These new "targeted agents" function like guided missiles that selectively home in on cancer cells while, at the same time, relatively sparing normal cells. These targeted therapies are already playing an important role in cancer treatment today, and most cancer experts predict that molecularly-targeted therapies will increasingly define the future of multidisciplinary cancer care (although these new molecular therapies are extraordinarily expensive at the present time).

For now, however, many cancer cells remain quite a bit smarter than we scientists and cancer physicians. Despite the recent development of novel new chemotherapy agents and molecularly-targeted drugs, cancer cells continue to demonstrate an amazing ability, over time, to eventually become resistant to these extremely expensive drugs by deploying various resistance or escape mechanisms. Unfortunately, we do not yet understand all of these complex and interrelated cancer cell escape mechanisms (for that matter, we still do not even completely understand all of the highly interconnected biochemical pathways present in normal cells, either). But the recent pace of scientific discovery in these areas has been truly astounding, and as we get closer to a more comprehensive understanding of the molecular biology of both normal cells and cancer cells, the hope is that we will eventually be able to simultaneously block multiple vital biochemical pathways in cancer cells. Using this multi-targeted approach, the hope is that cancer cells can be killed more quickly and more efficiently, and before they have a chance to mutate further and develop into treatment-resistant tumors (and all the while sparing most of the "innocent bystander" normal cells throughout the body).

Radiation Therapy

Radiation therapy, like chemotherapy, is typically used as a secondary, or adjuvant, form of cancer treatment for many types of solid tumors. Radiation therapy has become increasingly sophisticated in recent years, and newer technologies now enable radiation therapists to focus radiation beams almost exclusively upon the tumor and immediately adjacent tissues, thus minimizing the exposure of normal surrounding organs and tissues to unnecessary radiation. In certain cancers, such as cancers of the esophagus and rectum, radiation therapy is often routinely combined with chemotherapy *before* surgery is performed, in an effort to shrink large or otherwise advanced tumors, and to reduce the risk of local recurrence after surgery. Radiation therapy is also commonly used as neoadjuvant therapy (treatment given *before* surgery) in patients with locally-advanced breast cancers and sarcomas (malignant tumors of the soft tissues and bone) in the hope that the affected breast or extremity can be salvaged with less radical surgery.

Radiation therapy is rarely used by itself as primary treatment, although it may be given alone to patients who have metastatic spread of their cancer to the bone, or to other organs, as palliative therapy. However, when given as palliative therapy, as with palliative surgery or palliative chemotherapy, the primary goal of palliative radiation therapy is the relief of pain and suffering, and not cure.

References

1. Cancer Facts & Figures 2009, The American Cancer Society.

2. *CA: A Cancer Journal for Clinicians* 2008, 58:71-96.

3. Jemal A, et al. Annual Report to the Nation on the Status of Cancer, 1975–2005, Featuring Trends in Lung Cancer, Tobacco Use, and Tobacco Control. *Journal of the National Cancer Institute* 2008; 100:1672-1694.

4. Smith BD, et al. Future of cancer incidence in the United States: Burdens upon an aging, changing nation. *Journal of Clinical Oncology* 2009; 27:2745-2746.

5. SEER (*Surveillance Epidemiology and End Results*) Cancer Statistics Review 1975-2005.

CHAPTER 3

DIET & CANCER RISK

The role of diet in the development of cancer is an enormously complex area of research, and much of the data within this huge field of clinical study remains inconsistent and contradictory, unfortunately. However, there is still a great deal of useful research data available that should be considered when developing a diet-based strategy to reduce your lifetime risk of cancer. While the overall link between diet and cancer risk may not be entirely clear at this time, there are some specific cancers where diet *clearly* appears to affect cancer risk.

Numerous public health research studies have suggested that certain dietary patterns may be associated with a reduction in the risk of certain types of cancer. Time and time again, cancer prevention studies have shown that the increased consumption of red meat, highly processed meats (including sausages and luncheon meats), and other sources of animal fats, are associated with a significantly increased risk of death from several types of cancer (as well as from cardiovascular disease). In one very large prospective public health study, the enormous NIH-AARP study, more than 350,000 men and women between the ages of 50 and 71 years enrolled between 1995 and 1996. This massive group of research volunteers, all of whom were clinically healthy when they entered into the study, was then prospectively followed for an average duration of about 11 years. All of these study participants underwent analysis of their diets, with particular attention to the intake of fruits, vegetables, whole grains, low-fat or non-fat dairy products, very lean meats and poultry, and other sources of fat. Study volunteers who regularly consumed the *least* amount of animal fat, and who simultaneously also consumed the greatest amount of fruits, vegetables, and whole grains, experienced a *significantly* lower risk of death from cancer and cardiovascular disease. Moreover, the researchers conducting this study assessed each volunteer for other non-diet risk factors for cancer and cardiovascular disease, and even when adjusting for these other risk factors, people who ate poorly over the course of this 11-year study were still *12 percent* more likely to die from cancer and cardiovascular disease when compared to the volunteers with the healthiest diets [1].

The role of diet in the prevention of cancers of the gastrointestinal (GI) tract appears to be particularly strong. Studies of research volunteers who adhere to the so-called Mediterranean Diet (including large amounts of fresh fruits and vegetables, nuts, and fish) have repeatedly revealed a significantly reduced risk of cancers of the lung, esophagus, breast, stomach, colon, and rectum. Indeed, at least one such public health study, performed in Italy, found that strict adherence to the Mediterranean Diet was associated with a whopping *50 percent decrease in the risk of GI tract cancers* [2].

The Mediterranean Diet is generally understood to include lots of fresh fruits and vegetables, and moderate amounts of nuts, fish, and healthy cooking oils (and canola oil and olive oil, in particular). At the same time, the Mediterranean diet substitutes herbs and spices for salt, and may also include a modest amount of red wine (however, I must point out that regular alcohol intake has been shown to increase the risk of cancers of the breast, esophagus, stomach, colon, rectum, liver, pancreas, lung, bladder, and kidney). Finally, *like all effective cancer prevention diets*, very little, if any, red meat and processed meats are consumed in the Mediterranean Diet.

Other recent and large prospective public health studies further confirm that there are fundamental lifestyle and dietary habits that are unequivocally associated with a decreased risk of developing cancer (and many of these same healthy lifestyle habits also reduce the risk of that other top killer, cardiovascular disease). One such study, the large European Prospective Investigation into Cancer and Nutrition-Potsdam Study, enrolled more than 23,000 clinically healthy German volunteers between the ages of 35 and 65 years. Four fundamental lifestyle and diet-based factors were confirmed by this very large prospective clinical research trial to be associated with dramatic decreases in the incidence of serious diseases, including cancer. After an average of 8 years of follow-up, the study participants who routinely observed these 4 lifestyle and dietary factors had a nearly *40 percent lower risk of developing cancer* during the relatively short duration of this study, when compared to study participants who did not observe any of these 4 healthy lifestyle factors. *The 4 factors that consistently cut cancer risk by almost 40 percent included never having smoked, not being obese (body mass index, or BMI, less than 30), engaging in robust physical activity for at least 3.5 hours per week; and maintaining a healthy diet rich in fresh fruits, vegetables, and whole grains.* (Once again, this study confirmed that one of the most important components of a healthy "anti-cancer" diet was a very low intake of meat and other sources of animal fats.) *In addition to a nearly 40 percent reduction in the risk of developing cancer, adherents of these 4 critical lifestyle and dietary habits also achieved an astounding 93 percent reduction in the risk of diabetes, an 81 percent decrease in the risk of heart attack, and a 50 percent decrease in the risk of stroke, when compared to people who observed none of these 4 critical healthy lifestyle factors. Overall, the participants in this very large public health study who followed these 4 critical lifestyle and dietary habits had a 78 percent lower risk of chronic serious diseases (including cancer) when compared to people who did not observe these 4 tenets of a healthy cancer prevention lifestyle* [3].

Another very large European public health study, conducted in northern Italy between 1983 and 2004, evaluated more than 20,000 cancer cases, along with 18,000 patients without cancer. In this study, *the Mediterranean Diet was associated with a 30 to 70 percent reduction in the risk of gastrointestinal (GI) tract cancers.* Fruits and vegetables containing flavonoids and resveratrol were also associated with a significant decrease in the risk of breast cancer, as well [4].

Clinical studies strongly linking a Mediterranean-style diet with a significantly decreased risk of cancer are not limited to European countries. A particularly large prospective public health study in the United States followed more than 76,000 adult women for an average of 12 years. Detailed dietary surveys were conducted at various intervals during this large epidemiological study. As has been observed in multiple European studies, a healthy diet, characterized by abundant intake of fruits, vegetables, nuts, fish, poultry and whole grains was associated with a *46 percent reduction in the risk of colon cancer* when compared to the women who consumed the typical Western diet (i.e., a diet rich in red meat and other animal fats, and poor in fruits, vegetables, nuts, and whole grains) [5].

Numerous other studies have also shown a link between the increased consumption of red meat and processed meats and cancer risk, including cancers of the esophagus, stomach, colon, rectum, pancreas, lung, breast, prostate, kidney, and bladder. At the same time, cancer risk appears to be *decreased* by a diet rich in fish and, to a somewhat lesser extent, by diets rich in poultry as well [6, 7].

Pancreatic cancer is one of the deadliest of all types of cancer. Nearly 45,000 new cases of pancreatic cancer were diagnosed in 2009 in the United States, and more than 35,000 patients died of pancreatic cancer during the same year.

At the time of diagnosis, the vast majority of patients with this terrible disease are already incurable, and the overall 5-year survival rate for this type of cancer remains a dismal 5 percent at this time. Even among the small minority of patients who are diagnosed with pancreas cancer at a relatively early stage, when the tumor is still grossly confined to the pancreas, the 5-year survival rate is still only in the 15 to 20 percent range.

The only possible hope for pancreatic cancer cure is very radical surgery, which is often followed by chemotherapy and radiation therapy. For most patients with pancreatic cancer, however, surgery is not even an option due to the advanced stage of their cancer at the time of diagnosis. Therefore, increased efforts to prevent pancreatic cancer are critically important in decreasing the death rate from this aggressive and treatment-resistant form of cancer.

There are several well-known risk factors for pancreatic cancer. These include smoking, obesity, diabetes, increased meat intake, chronic pancreatitis (inflammation of the pancreas), and chronic liver disease. Because of the known links between pancreatic cancer and diabetes, and obesity as well, there is also concern that the frequent consumption of foods that significantly elevate the level of glucose (sugar) in the blood may also increase the risk of developing pancreatic cancer.

In one large prospective public health study with a long duration of follow-up, nearly 61,000 patient volunteers within the Singapore Chinese Health Study were followed for up to 14 years by researchers. All of these volunteers were extensively surveyed regarding their consumption of juices, sugary sodas ("soft drinks"), and other dietary items. Additionally, other lifestyle factors and environmental exposures linked to various types of cancer were assessed within this very large group of patients.

Over a 14-year period, 140 new cases of pancreatic cancer were diagnosed within this very large cohort of patient volunteers. When the researchers analyzed all of this study's data, they discovered that the consumption of 2 or more sugary sodas per week was associated with nearly *twice* the risk of developing pancreatic cancer when compared to not drinking any sodas at all (fortunately, there appeared to be no link between juice intake and pancreatic cancer risk) [8].

The findings of this study add further evidence to previous similar studies regarding the intake of so-called "high glycemic index" foods and pancreatic cancer risk. As these same sugar-rich foods also directly contribute to the development of both diabetes and obesity, it is not surprising that scientists have begun to identify common biochemical pathways that link excessive calorie intake from sugar-rich foods with all three of these life-threatening diseases.

Based upon this study, and others like it, if you currently drink sodas containing the sugars sucrose or fructose on a regular basis, you might want to seriously consider eliminating these soft drinks from your diet altogether.

Another recently published study, from Italy, compared 326 pancreatic cancer patients with 652 matched "control patients" without pancreatic cancer. In this study, the regular addition of table sugar (sucrose) to foods and beverages was also found to *more than double the risk* of pancreatic cancer. The frequent consumption of potatoes, which are associated with a moderate "glycemic load," also appeared to *almost double* the risk of pancreatic cancer. As has been demonstrated in many other previous research studies, the frequent consumption of meat (and red meat and processed meats, in particular) was also associated with a *doubling of pancreatic cancer risk*, as well. At the same time, this public health study found that regularly eating fresh non-citrus fruits and vegetables appeared to *cut the risk of this deadly cancer in half* [9].

There is a large body of public health research data linking the frequent consumption of fresh fruits and vegetables with a lower risk of some types of cancer. In fact, there is compelling research evidence that an apple a day may do much more than just "keep the doctor away." According to a recently published hospital-based clinical study that included 592 patients with colorectal cancer and 765 patients without any history of cancer, colorectal cancer patients consumed less fruit than patients without cancer (9.5 servings per week versus 11 servings per week, respectively). Based upon detailed dietary surveys conducted by experienced interviewers, the two groups of patients differed mostly in the number of apples that they regularly consumed, which accounted for 80 percent of the observed difference in fruit intake between the two groups of patient volunteers. *In this small dietary survey-based study, the consumption of one apple per day was associated with a 35 percent reduction in the risk of developing colorectal cancer, while eating 2 or more apples per day appeared to reduce the risk of colorectal cancer by about 50 percent.* The authors surmised that flavonoids, and other polyphenols, contained in red apples may explain the observed reduction in colorectal cancer risk associated with eating apples [10]. (While this is a rather small and low-powered study, its findings have been mirrored in other larger and more powerful studies, although the total risk reduction for colorectal cancer observed in other larger studies has not been as dramatic as was noted in this particular hospital-based study.)

References

1. Kant AK, et al. Patterns of recommended dietary behaviors predict subsequent risk of mortality in a large cohort of men and women in the United States. *Journal of Nutrition* 2009; 139:1374-1380.

2. La Vecchia C, Boestti C. Diet and cancer risk in Mediterranean countries: open issues. *Public Health Nutrition* 2006; 9:1077-1082.

3. Ford ES, et al. Healthy living is the best revenge. *Archives of Internal Medicine* 2009; 169:1355-1362.

4. La Vecchia C, Boestti C. Diet and cancer risk in Mediterranean countries: open issues. *Public Health Nutrition* 2006; 9:1077-1082.

5. Fung T, Hu FB, Fuchs C, et al. Major dietary patterns and the risk of colorectal cancer in women. *Archives of Internal Medicine* 2003, 163:309-314.]

6. Hu J, et al. Meat and fish consumption and cancer in Canada. *Nutrition & Cancer* 2008; 50:313-324.

7. Fernandez E, et al. Fish consumption and cancer risk. *American Journal of Clinical Nutrition* 1999; 70:85-90.

8. Mueller NT, et al. Soft drink and juice consumption and risk of pancreatic cancer: the Singapore Chinese Health Study. *Cancer Epidemiology, Biomarkers & Prevention* 2010; 19:447-455

9. Polesel J, et al. Dietary habits and risk of pancreatic cancer: an Italian case-control study. *Cancer Causes & Control* 2009 [Epub ahead of print].

10. Jedrychowski W, et al. Case-control study on beneficial effect of regular consumption of apples on colorectal cancer risk in a population with relatively low intake of fruits and vegetables. *European Journal of Cancer Prevention* 2010; 19;42-47.

CHAPTER 4

ALCOHOL AND CANCER RISK

The data linking increased and regular alcohol intake to the risk of multiple forms of cancer is both abundant and persuasive. For example, the Million Women Study, one of the largest prospective epidemiological studies ever undertaken, recruited nearly 1.3 million middle-aged women who were followed for more than 7 years, on average. Alcohol consumption by these women was then correlated with the incidence of new cancers that were diagnosed during the course of this massive public health study. For every increase in the average number of daily alcohol drinks, there was a 29 percent increase in the relative risk of oral cavity cancer, a 44 percent increase in the relative risk of laryngeal cancer, a 22 percent increase in the relative risk of esophageal cancer, a 10 percent increase in the relative risk of rectal cancer, a 24 percent increase in the relative risk of liver cancer, a 12 percent increase in the relative risk of breast cancer, and a 6 percent increase in total cancer relative risk (the risk of oral cavity and laryngeal cancer was only increased by alcohol intake in smokers, however). It is important to point out that these increased cancer risks were observed for *all* types of alcoholic beverages, including wine [1].

Yet another clinical study, from Canada, also linked regular alcohol intake with an increased risk of several specific types of cancer, including cancers of the esophagus, stomach, colon, liver, pancreas and lung [2].

While all patients should be advised to moderate their alcohol intake, women, in particular, need to be aware that there are multiple clinical research studies confirming a significant link between regular alcohol intake and breast cancer risk. Indeed, a recent meta-analysis, based on data from 53 different clinical research studies, concluded that alcohol *increased the relative risk of developing breast cancer by 7 percent for each daily single serving of alcohol consumed.* Furthermore, the results from this large meta-analysis study suggest that about 4 *percent of all breast cancers* in developed countries may be caused directly by alcohol consumption. Finally, this landmark study found that *even a single alcoholic beverage per day* was associated with a statistically significant *increase* in the risk of developing breast cancer [3].

References

1.   Allen NE, et al. Moderate alcohol intake and cancer incidence in women. *Journal of the National Cancer Institute* 2009; 101:296-305.

2.   Benedetti A, et al. Lifetime consumption of alcoholic beverages and risk of 13 types of cancer in men: results from a case-control study in Montreal. *Cancer Detection & Prevention* 2009; 32:352-362.

3.   Mahoney MC, et al. Opportunities and Strategies for Breast Cancer Prevention Through Risk Reduction. *CA, A Cancer Journal for Clinicians* 2008; 58:347-371.

CHAPTER 5

OBESITY & CANCER RISK

Undoubtedly, our ancient ancestors lived a rather harsh existence compared to our lives in the modern world, today. Nutritional needs were not met, thousands of years ago, by bringing home groceries from the local supermarket, or by stopping at a favorite nearby restaurant. And so, we appear to have evolved, biologically, to hoard and ingest high-calorie foods whenever the opportunity to do so presents itself. Ten thousand years ago, the occasional success of bands of nomadic hunters in felling a large animal meant that the tribe would go to sleep with full bellies that night. Today, however, we live in a world with an overabundance of highly processed foods that are stuffed with supra-normal levels of calories and fat. Most of us also live in a world where we are surrounded by effort-saving convenience devices, including cars and other means of conveyance, electronic remote control devices, elevators, escalators, and all manner of other powered devices that markedly decrease our daily activity levels.

Our preferred forms of entertainment have also radically changed over even the past five or six decades. Instead of engaging in sports and recreational activities like hiking, running, climbing, swimming, rowing, or other calorie-burning physical activities, we now plop ourselves down on sofas and cushy recliners and watch television, or a movie, or a concert, or *other* people playing sports, for hours at a time. Therefore, we burn *fewer calories* each day than any society in history. Meanwhile, we consume *more calories* than any other culture or civilization before us. Thus, it shouldn't be surprising that obesity has truly become an epidemic in the United States, and throughout much of the world. In the United States, for example, an astounding *68 percent of all adults are either overweight or obese, while 34 percent are obese, and at least 2 percent of the adult population is considered "morbidly obese"* [1].

Even the most conservative estimates have predicted that as many as 40 percent of all cancer cases, and more than 30 percent of all cancer deaths, could be prevented by relatively simple changes in diet and physical activity levels, alone. Thus far, the cancers that have been particularly linked to excessive body weight include cancers of the esophagus, colon, rectum, liver, gallbladder, pancreas, kidney, stomach (at least in men), prostate, breast, uterus, cervix, and ovary. Being overweight or obese has been estimated to directly account for 14 percent of all cancers in men and 20 percent of all cancers in women. Thus, it has been estimated that the adoption of prudent dietary and related lifestyle measures would dramatically decrease the incidence of obesity-associated cancers, including an estimated 60 to 70 percent reduction in the risk of cancers of the breast, prostate, colon, and rectum [2, 3]. For example, in a recently published case-control study by the American Cancer Society, 1,794 patients with newly diagnosed colorectal cancer and 2,684 of their same-sex siblings without colorectal cancer were analyzed. In this study, rising levels of obesity were significantly correlated to increased colorectal cancer risk in both men and women [4].

Based upon data compiled by the American Institute for Cancer Research and the American Cancer Society, excess body fat is estimated to cause at least 100,500 new cases of cancer every year in the United States, including:

49%	of endometrial cancers	(20,700 cases/year)
35%	of esophageal cancers	(5,800 cases/year)
28%	of pancreatic cancers	(11,900 cases/year)
24%	of kidney cancers	(13, 900 cases/year)
21%	of gallbladder cancers	(2,000 cases/year)
17%	of breast cancers	(33,000 cases/year)
9%	of colorectal cancers	(13,200 cases/year)

[American Institute for Cancer Research/WCRF's Policy and Action for Cancer Prevention, 2009; Cancer Facts and Figures 2009, American Cancer Society]

Therefore, based upon conservative estimates, at least 100,000 cases of cancer could be prevented each year in the United States, alone, simply by avoiding excess body weight. (*These 100,000 preventable cases of cancer represent 7 percent of all cases of cancers that were diagnosed in the United States in 2009.*) Thus, even without drastically altering our lifestyle in other ways, we can drive down our risk of cancer by almost 10 percent, simply by maintaining a normal body weight (BMI < 25) [5]!

(I will discuss the impact of obesity on breast and prostate cancer risk in the chapters dedicated to these two cancers, later in this book.)

References

1. Flegal KM, et al. Prevalence and trends in obesity among US adults, 1999-2008. *Journal of the American Medical Association* 2010; 303:235-241.

2. Donaldson MS. Nutrition and cancer: a review of the evidence for an anti-cancer diet. *Nutrition Journal* 2004; 3:19.

3. Cancer Facts & Figures 2009, American Cancer Society.

4. Campbell PT, et al. Case-control study of overweight, obesity, and colorectal cancer risk, overall and by tumor microsatellite instability status. *Journal of the National Cancer Institute* 2010; 102:391-400.

5. Cancer Facts & Figures 2009, American Cancer Society

CHAPTER 6

STRESS & CANCER RISK

We live in a stressful world. As I write this book, the United States, and much of the world, is struggling to emerge from the worst economic recession in more than 70 years. Unemployment is high, and taxes are rising. The deficit in America, and in other countries as well, has already far surpassed the level that economists believe is sustainable. An extreme polarization of views permeates both the government and society in the United States, and in many other countries around the world. War, hunger, natural disasters, global warming, crime, and myriad other plagues and crises fill our daily lives with stress and worry.

There is ample research data showing that chronic levels of increased stress raise the risk of cardiovascular disease, but what about the impact of chronic stress on our risk of developing cancer? (The constant surveillance of our immune system for abnormal cells is one of the body's most important defenses against cancer, and chronic stress is known to impair immune function. Moreover, it has long been known that organ transplant patients have a much higher risk of developing certain types of cancer as a result of having their immune systems suppressed with anti-rejection drugs.) However, the research data available is, at best, mixed with respect to chronic stress and cancer risk.

Perhaps the most influential recent public health study linking severe stress with cancer risk is a *retrospective* study of Israeli Jewish survivors of World War II. In this study, more than 250,000 Israeli Jews who remained in Europe during World War II were compared with more than 55,000 Israeli Jews who emigrated from Europe before or during World War II. The incidence of cancer in these two very large groups of World War II survivors was then assessed using a national cancer registry. This study found that Jewish people who remained in Europe during World War II had a significantly *higher* risk of cancer, and a *higher risk of colorectal cancer and breast cancer in particular.* Among the Jewish men who remained in Europe throughout World War II (as children, of course), the *relative* risk of cancer was *almost 4 times greater* than was observed in the group of Jewish men who left Europe before or during World War II. Likewise, the *relative* risk of cancer was more than *2 times greater* among the Jewish women who remained in Europe throughout the War, when compared to the women who left before or during the War. However, this study has been heavily criticized because it *infers* that the Jewish men and women who remained in Europe throughout World War II, as children, were *all* subjected to more physical and emotional stress, whereas those who left before or during the War experienced less stress. As the authors of this study were not able to identify which among these more than 300,000 Jews had directly fallen victim to the Holocaust, the division of this large cohort of Jewish men and women into these two groups is somewhat arbitrary. Therefore, the conclusion that Israeli Jews *potentially exposed to the Holocaust* had a higher incidence of cancer due to stress cannot be proven by this particular study, although the findings of this innovative study are quite intriguing [1].

A large prospective public health study from Baltimore has suggested that chronic depression may be associated with an increased risk of cancer. In this study, 3,177 adults were prospectively followed for an average of 24 years, during which 334 cases of cancer were diagnosed. After adjusting for other cancer risk factors, patients with a formal diagnosis of depression in this study were found to have *2 times the risk* of developing cancer when compared to the study volunteers who had never been diagnosed with depression. Among the patient volunteers with depression, the risk of developing breast cancer, specifically, was *4 times greater* than what was observed among the volunteers without a history of depression. Depression also appeared to increase the risk of prostate cancer, as well, but this finding did not quite reach statistical significance [2].

Another study, a meta-analysis of 13 prospective public health studies, found that the risk of breast cancer was almost *3 times higher* among chronically depressed women when compared to women without a history of depression (although, interestingly, only the evaluated studies that followed patient volunteers for 10 or more years revealed this apparent link between depression and breast cancer risk). No associations between depression and cancers of the lung, prostate, colon or rectum were identified in this study, however [3].

At the same time, other public health studies have failed to identify a link between chronic stress and cancer risk. For example, more than 11,000 women who participated in the landmark European Prospective Investigation into Cancer (EPIC) prospective clinical research study were followed for an average of 10 years. Comprehensive surveys were used to assess childhood and adult stress levels and adverse events. Over a 10-year period, 313 new cases of breast cancer were diagnosed in this large group of women. Following a comprehensive assessment of lifetime social adversity for all of these patient volunteers, no association was found between chronic stress levels and breast cancer risk [4].

In summary, while the available research data does not strongly appear to support a direct link between chronic stress and overall cancer risk, some "observational" public health studies have suggested a possible link between stress (and depression) and cancer risk. As our immune system plays an important role in cancer surveillance and prevention, it is conceivable that chronic stress might be a potential risk factor for cancer, including breast cancer.

References

1. Krinasn-Boker L. et al. Cancer incidence in Israeli Jewish survivors of World War II. *Journal of the National Cancer Institute* 2009; 101:1489-1500.

2. Gross AL, et al. Depression and cancer risk: 24 years of follow-up of the Baltimore Epidemiologic Catchment Area sample. *Cancer Epidemiology* 2010; 21:191-199.

3. Oerlemans ME, et al. A meta-analysis on depression and subsequent cancer risk. *Clinical Practice and Epidemiology in Mental Health* 2007; 3:29.

4. Surtees PG, et al. No evidence that social stress is associated with breast cancer incidence. *Breast Cancer Research & Incidence* 2010; 120;169-174.

CHAPTER 7

DIABETES & CANCER RISK

It is becoming increasingly apparent that diabetes is a significant risk factor for cancer. For example, the enormous Nurses' Health Study, which included approximately 120,000 women volunteers between the ages of 30 and 55 years, found that diabetes was associated with a *43 percent increase* in the *relative* risk of colon cancer, and an *11 percent increase* in the *relative* risk of rectal cancer. Diabetic women were also far more likely to develop advanced and fatal colorectal cancers when compared to women without diabetes [1].

In addition to an increased risk of colorectal cancer, diabetes is known to increase the risk of one of the deadliest forms of cancer, pancreatic cancer, by as much as *50 percent* [2]. Other studies have suggested that diabetes may also be associated with an increased risk of cancers of the breast, liver, kidney, and uterus, in addition to the colon, rectum and pancreas. (Oddly enough, diabetes may *decrease* the risk of developing prostate cancer.) There is also compelling evidence that diabetic patients who maintain excellent control of their diabetes can significantly reduce their risk of developing cancer [3-5].

References

1. Hu FB, et al. Prospective study of adult onset diabetes mellitus (type 2) and risk of colorectal cancer in women. *Journal of the National Cancer Institute* 1999; 17:542-547.

2. Gioavannucci E, Michaud D. The role of obesity and related metabolic disturbances in cancers of the colon, prostate, and pancreas. *Gastroenterology* 2007; 132:2208-2225.

3.   Vigneri P, et al. Diabetes and cancer. *Endocrine-Related Cancer* 2009; 16:1103-1123.

4.   Ogunleye AA, et al. A cohort study of the risk of cancer associated with type 2 diabetes. *British Journal of Cancer* 2009; 101:1199-1201.

5.   Zhang Y, et al. The association between metabolic abnormality and endometrial cancer: a large case-control study in China. *Gynecologic Oncology* 2010 [Epub ahead of print].

CHAPTER 8

ENVIRONMENTAL FACTORS & CANCER RISK

Air Pollution and Cancer

Man-made particulate pollutants are primarily generated from the combustion of fossil fuels and wood products. The most common sources of cancer-causing air pollutants include coal-burning power plants, diesel engines, and wood-burning. In addition to an increased risk of lung cancer associated with chronic exposure to particulate air pollution, cancers of the GI tract, bladder, and female genital tract, as well as leukemia, have also been linked to increased air pollution exposure. By at least one estimate, 5 percent of male cancer deaths in the United States, and 3 percent of female cancer deaths, can be attributed to particulate air pollution exposure [1, 2].

High-Voltage Power Lines and Cancer

There has been an ongoing debate, for more than three decades now, regarding the potential effects of high-voltage power lines on cancer risk. Concerns about power lines and cancer risk arose after several low-powered public health studies reported an apparent clustering of cases of leukemia and lymphoma among children in neighborhoods adjacent to high-voltage power line towers [3, 4]. Unfortunately, it remains unclear, at this time, whether or not electromagnetic fields (EMFs) from high-voltage power lines can induce cancer (in either children or adults), as establishing a direct cause-and-effect relationship is nearly impossible. (Moreover, most of the published research studies linking EMFs to an increased risk of cancer have been seriously flawed.) In general, however, as there still remains some uncertainty regarding a possible association between chronic exposure to EMFs and cancer risk, it is probably best to avoid prolonged exposure to nearby high-tension power lines, particularly for babies and children.

Cell Phones & Microwaves

There has been considerable concern regarding a potential link between mobile cell phone use and the development of both benign and malignant brain tumors. Because it is so difficult to establish a direct link between cell phone use and brain tumors, most of the published clinical research data in this area has been developed from relatively low-powered research studies. Therefore, meta-analysis studies, which combine multiple relatively low-powered studies to create a more powerful "meta-study," can be helpful in the absence of large high-powered research studies. One such meta-analysis, from Korea, analyzed 23 case-control studies that, altogether, included nearly 40,000 volunteers. When the results of *all 23 studies* were considered, cell phone use did *not* appear to increase the risk of either benign or malignant brain tumors. However, when only *the 13 highest quality* clinical studies were evaluated by meta-analysis, the results became more concerning, as an apparent *18 percent increase* in the risk of brain tumors associated with cell phone use was identified [5].

Another meta-analysis, from Sweden, found that 10 or more years of cell phone use was associated with a significantly increased risk of brain tumors, as well [6].

Thus, there is some clinical research data available to suggest that the long-term use of cell phones *may* be associated with an increased risk of benign and malignant brain tumors, although the research data is not uniformly consistent in this area. However, there remains enough concern regarding a potential link between cell phone use and brain tumor risk that I believe it is prudent to minimize the use of mobile cell phones. Whether or not the use of "hands-free" devices decreases any apparent brain tumor risk that might be associated with frequent cell phone use is unknown at this time. However, keeping cell phones as far away from one's head as possible will significantly reduce the amount of microwave radiation that is transmitted from the phone's antenna to the brain. As multiple studies have shown a dose-dependent and time-dependent effect of cell phone exposure on the apparent risk of brain tumors, increasing the distance between cell phones and the brain, and reducing the overall use of cell phones to a minimum, may decrease the risk of brain tumors. Once again, I must stress that there is conflicting data regarding the potential health effects of cell phones on the human brain. However, there is enough data available to remain concerned, especially given the frequent and pervasive use of these devices throughout the world.

Cell phones are not the only source of environmental microwave radiation exposure. Cordless telephones, microwave ovens, and microwave transmission and relay towers are other common environmental sources of microwave exposure. At this time, however, there is no solid research evidence available suggesting that exposure to typical environmental levels of microwave radiation is associated with a significantly increased risk of cancer.

Solar Radiation & Tanning Beds

Exposure to the sun's ultraviolet rays is a known risk factor for the three most common types of skin cancer (basal cell cancer, squamous cell cancer, and melanoma). The use of tanning beds, which sharply increases ultraviolet radiation exposure, is also a recognized risk factor for skin cancer. (Fair-skinned people are at particularly increased risk of developing skin cancer secondary to chronic sun exposure.)

While basal cell and squamous cell skin cancers rarely spread (metastasize) to other areas of the body, melanoma can rapidly and extensively spread to almost any organ in the body if it is not detected and treated early enough. In addition to a family history of melanoma, frequent blistering sunburns during childhood and adolescence have also been clearly linked with an increased lifetime risk of melanoma. Additionally, having a large number of pigmented moles (nevi) is also a known risk factor for melanoma [7].

Diagnostic X-rays

It has recently been estimated that up to *2 percent of all cancer* cases are directly caused by exposure to medical x-ray tests. Although most radiation experts believe that there is no completely safe level of exposure to x-rays, it is well known that exposure to increasing doses of x-rays, as well as undergoing repeated x-ray examinations, increases the overall risk of cancer formation.

Clinical data from the World War II atomic bombings in Japan, and from the more recent Chernobyl nuclear reactor accident in 1986, provide the most comprehensive clinical data available regarding the effects of large radiation doses on cancer risk in humans. (The extensive long-term epidemiological data arising from the atomic bombings in Japan has been used as the primary benchmark with which to assess the potential impact of diagnostic x-ray examinations on cancer risk in humans.) Even more than 6 decades following the 1945 atomic bombings in Hiroshima and Nagasaki, the incidence of cancer among bomb survivors continues to rise. The cancers that have been most specifically linked to exposure to even low doses of atomic bomb fall-out are leukemia, lymphoma (a cancer of the lymph nodes), thyroid cancer, stomach cancer, lung cancer, liver cancer, bladder cancer, and uterine cancer.

Although the duration of follow-up from the Chernobyl nuclear disaster is still rather limited, a significant increase in the risk of thyroid cancer has already been confirmed across the swath of Europe downwind from the breached reactor core [8, 9].

Outside of radiation therapy treatments for cancer, CT (computed tomography) scans have become the most common source of clinical exposure to ionizing radiation. CT scanners have, unquestionably, revolutionized the practice of medicine since they were first introduced into routine clinical practice in 1974. CT scanners utilize a rotating x-ray device to create hundreds of individual images that can then be reconstructed by computers into a complex three dimensional view of the body. Current generation CT scanners are able to image the entire human body within seconds, and these high definition images provide physicians with an incredibly detailed view of the organs and tissues deep within our bodies

CT scanners have become a virtually indispensible diagnostic tool within almost every medical and surgical specialty, and an estimated 75 million CT scans are now performed annually in the United States, alone. As the popularity of these complex and powerful diagnostic imaging machines has continued to grow, so has the frequency of their use for clinically dubious reasons. For example, routine scans of the heart, and its coronary arteries, have, increasingly, been used for "screening purposes" in patients without any clinical evidence of heart disease. Likewise, there has been an explosion in the number of private radiology imaging centers offering fee-based "body scans" for clinically healthy people who are interested in having their internal organs examined for early signs of diseases that can be detected by CT scans. Another area of concern regarding the use of CT scanners is that physicians have become so dependent on these machines, and the exquisite images of the human body that they provide, that many (if not most) doctors have a very low threshold to order CT scans as a routine part of their diagnostic work-up of patients. (For example, in my own specialty of Surgery, the diagnosis of appendicitis is now routinely made with a CT scanner, rather than by the traditional method of a surgeon's clinical evaluation of the patient.)

While CT scanners have become essential diagnostic tools, they also expose patients to much higher doses of radiation than most conventional x-ray examinations. Moreover, there has been a growing concern regarding the actual dose of radiation that is being delivered to patients from CT scanners across the country, as there is a great deal of variability in the radiation dose settings being used at different CT scan imaging facilities. This alarming point was recently brought to the public's attention when it was revealed that Cedars Sinai Medical Center, a prestigious private teaching hospital in the Beverly Hills area, was being investigated after multiple patients who had undergone CT scans of their brain there began to notice that their hair was falling out. Authorities subsequently determined that these patients had received grossly excessive radiation doses during their CT scans.

Two recently published clinical research studies on radiation doses associated with routine CT scans have strongly suggested that the experiences of patients at Cedars Sinai Medical Center may not be uncommon, unfortunately.

The first of these two studies quantified the amount of radiation dose delivered to 1,119 patients during 11 common types of CT scan examinations that were performed at 4 different hospitals in the San Francisco area. In addition to calculating the radiation doses received by these patients, the authors also estimated the probable lifetime cancer risk associated with these CT scans. As the Cedars Sinai case has already shown, there appears to be considerable variability in the amount of radiation exposure used at different institutions to conduct the same exact type of CT scan. However, the sheer magnitude of this variability in radiation doses, as measured by these researchers, is both mind-boggling and disturbing. Not only was there an enormous difference in radiation doses associated with performing the same exact type of CT scan *between* the 4 different institutions that were studied, but significant radiation exposure differences were also present *within each individual institution when performing the same type of CT scan examination on different patients!* When the researchers had finished their calculations, they noted an almost unbelievable *13-fold difference*, on average, in radiation exposure for the same type of CT scan (from the highest to the lowest observed radiation doses) performed on different patients.

Based upon cancer incidence data collected after the Hiroshima and Nagasaki atomic bombings, this study's researchers calculated that an estimated *1 in 270 women* who underwent CT scans of their coronary arteries at age 40 will eventually develop cancer as a direct result of these CT scans (versus *1 in 600 men*), while *1 in 8,100 women* who underwent CT scans of the brain at age 40 will develop cancer from these scans (versus *1 in 11,080 men*). For men and women who underwent CT scans at age 20 (instead of age 40), the projected lifetime risk of CT scan-associated cancer was *nearly double* the projected risk of the 40 year-old patients [10].

The findings of this study indicate that the variability in radiation exposure between hospitals for the same type of CT scan examination is much greater than was previously believed. Perhaps even more surprising was the finding that identical CT scan examinations performed within a single hospital also subjected patients to significantly differing amounts of radiation exposure. Finally, the calculated range of radiation exposure for CT scans revealed that, in general, *patients are receiving far higher doses of radiation from routine CT scans than has generally been appreciated.* (For example, a single CT coronary artery angiogram delivers the same amount of radiation as *310 chest x-rays!*)

The second (and related) research study used public health data to estimate the average number of radiation-induced cancers caused by CT scans throughout the United States. Based upon current CT scan utilization across the country, these researchers predicted that, in the United States alone, approximately 29,000 future cases of cancer, and 15,000 cancer-associated deaths, could be expected to arise from CT scans performed in 2007, alone [11].

Other clinical studies have estimated that repetitive CT scans of the body, over the course of a person's lifetime, might result in as much as a *2 percent lifetime risk* of dying from cancer as a direct result of such scans. In fact, even a *single* whole-body CT scan has been estimated, in one study, to produce a 0.08 percent lifetime risk of dying due to a radiation-induced cancer [12]!

These studies are real eye-openers that should cause all of us, physicians and patients alike, to reconsider the benefits versus the risks of each and every CT scan that is considered before such scans are ordered. Although most CT scans are performed because they offer vitally important clinical information, numerous CT scans are still being ordered and performed for far less compelling reasons (one of them being, unquestionably, the tendency of many physicians to order multiple unnecessary tests on patients as part of their practice of "defensive medicine"). Moreover, the striking variation in CT-associated radiation doses, and the unexpectedly high level of these radiation doses in general, points to the need to improve standardization and compliance at every one of the thousands of institutions in the United States that operates a CT scanner. Meanwhile, a higher threshold for ordering CT scans is important, as is the greater use (when appropriate) of ultrasound and magnetic resonance imaging (MRI) scans in place of CT scans.

Therapeutic Radiation

Radiation therapy is an indispensible part of cancer treatment, and many lives are prolonged, or saved, thanks to modern radiation therapy. However, as with exposure to other forms of ionizing radiation, radiation therapy is (ironically) associated with a small but significant increase in the lifetime risk of developing cancer. For example, breast cancer and lymphoma patients who have previously received therapeutic radiation therapy to the chest are at increased lifelong risk of developing lung cancer, with radiation-induced lung cancers arising, on average, 5 to 10 years following completion of radiation therapy.

One of the most intensively studied examples of cancer associated with radiation therapy is the increased incidence of breast cancer among women who were treated with radiation to the chest for Hodgkin's lymphoma during childhood or adolescence. In one of the largest and most comprehensive studies of female Hodgkin's disease patients, the risk of developing breast cancer among women who received higher doses of radiation to the chest area ranges *from 3 to 8 times the incidence* observed in patients who received very low radiation doses to the chest [13].

Radiation treatment to the pelvis for prostate cancer has also been linked to an increased risk of subsequent rectal and bladder cancers. In one study, using a large national cancer database in the United States, more than 250,000 prostate cancer cases were reviewed and analyzed. The risk of subsequent bladder cancer was *nearly twice as common* (or 100 percent more common) among the men who received external beam radiation therapy for their prostate cancer when compared to men who underwent surgical removal of their prostate glands. The incidence of rectal cancer was also noted to be *1.2 times more common* (or 20 percent more common) among the prostate cancer patients who received external beam radiation therapy instead of surgery [14].

(Of note, the increased risk of secondary bladder cancer was less when brachytherapy, or "radioactive seed" therapy, was used as radiation therapy, and brachytherapy of the prostate gland did not appear to increase the risk of rectal cancer in this study.)

All cancer experts agree that, when used properly, the health benefits of modern radiation therapy significantly outweigh the risks. The recent development of new radiation delivery technologies, including "conformal radiation," in which the targeting and dosing of radiation beams concentrates almost all of the radiation dose on the tumor and the immediately surrounding tissues and organs, should help to reduce radiation doses to "innocent bystander" tissues and organs and, hopefully, will further reduce the risk of secondary cancers induced by radiation treatments.

Radon Gas

Chronic exposure to radon gas is the second most common risk factor for lung cancer, and as with other non-tobacco lung cancer risk factors, smokers who are chronically exposed to radon gas have an even greater risk of developing lung cancer than similarly exposed non-smokers.

Radon is a colorless, odorless and tasteless radioactive gas that results from the natural isotopic decay of uranium. (Uranium is ubiquitously present, in varying concentrations, within the bedrock beneath the soil.) Radon gas easily seeps through tiny cracks in basement foundations and walls, and closed spaces in buildings at or below ground level can trap radon gas until it reaches concentrations that are high enough to induce lung cancer. Published scientific estimates regarding the percentage of lung cancer cases caused by radon gas exposure vary, but it is generally agreed that 5 to 10 percent of all lung cancer cases are directly caused by radon gas.

Other Environmental Cancer Risk Factors

In addition to radon gas and other sources of ionizing radiation, environmental exposures to increased levels of asbestos, nickel, cobalt, cadmium, chromium, and diesel exhaust have also been implicated in the development of lung cancer. Moreover, smoking appears to have an additive, or synergistic, cancer-causing effect when combined with exposure to asbestos, radon gas, and uranium ore. Although the precise contribution of each of these potential environmental carcinogens to the overall incidence of lung cancer is not completely understood, they are thought to account for only a very small percentage of all lung cancer cases diagnosed in the United States. Smoking and radon gas, on the other hand, account for 95 to 99 percent of all lung cancer cases in the United States, and throughout the world as well.

References

1. Grant WB. Air pollution in relation to U.S. cancer mortality rates: an ecological study; likely role of carbonaceous aerosols and polycyclic aromatic hydrocarbons. *Anticancer Research* 2009; 29:3537-3545.

2. Beelen R, et al. Long-term exposure to traffic-related air pollution and lung cancer risk. *Epidemiology* 2008; 19:702-710.

3. Draper G, et al. Childhood cancer in relation to distance from high voltage power lines in England and Wales: a case control study. *British Medical Journal* 2005; 330:1290.

4. Lowenthal RM, et al. Residential exposure to electric power transmission lines and risk of lymphoproliferative and myeloproliferative disorders: a case-control study. *Internal Medicine Journal* 2007; 37:614-619.

5. Myung SK, et al. Mobile phone use and risk of tumors: a meta-analysis. *Journal of Clinical Oncology* 2009; 27:5565-5572.

6. Hardell L. et al. Meta-analysis of long-term mobile phone use and the association with brain tumors. *International Journal of Oncology* 2008; 32:1097-1103.

7. Naldi L, et al. Sun exposure, phenotypic characteristics, and cutaneous malignant melanoma. An analysis according to different clinical-pathological variant and anatomic locations (Italy). *Cancer Causes & Control* 2005; 16:893-899.

8. Dropkin G. Reanalysis of cancer mortality in Japanese A-bomb survivors exposed to low doses of radiation: bootstrap and simulation methods. *Environmental Health* 2009; 9:56.

9. Cardis E, et al. Estimates of the cancer burden in Europe from radioactive fallout from the Chernobul accident. *International Journal of Cancer* 2005; 119:1224-12235.

10. Smith-Bindman R, et al. Radiation dose associated with common computed tomography examination and the associated lifetime attributable risk of cancer. *Archives of Internal Medicine* 2009; 169:2078-2086.

11. Berrington de González A, et al. Projected cancer risks from computed tomographic scans performed in the United States in 2007. *Archives of Internal Medicine 2009*; 169:2071-2077.

12. Brenner DJ, Elliston CD. Estimated radiation risks potentially associated with full-body CT screening. *Radiology* 2004; 232:735-738.

13. Travis LB, et al. Breast cancer following radiotherapy and chemotherapy among young women with Hodgkin disease. *Journal of the American Medical Association* 2003; 290:465-475.

14. Nieder AM, et al. Radiation therapy for prostate cancer increases subsequent risk of bladder and rectal cancer: a population based cohort study. *Journal of Urology* 2008; 180:2005-2009.

CHAPTER 9

INFECTION & CANCER RISK

Helicobacter pylori

Chronic infections with so-called "oncogenic" (cancer-causing) viruses and bacteria can lead to a variety of cancers. Most of these oncogenic organisms can either be prevented by vaccines, or effectively eliminated with antibiotics. The contribution of these viral and bacterial infections to the overall cancer burden among humans is striking, and is inadequately appreciated.

An estimated two-thirds of the world's population is chronically infected with a bacterium known as *Helicobacter pylori*. This peculiarly curved bacterium is highly specialized to live in the human stomach, and is a common cause of inflammatory illnesses of the stomach and small intestine, including gastritis, gastric (stomach) ulcers, and duodenal ulcers.

The story behind the discovery of *H. pylori* as a cause of chronic inflammation and ulcers of the stomach and duodenum is a fascinating one. When *H. pylori* was initially discovered in the lining of the stomach and duodenum of patients with ulcers, in the early 1980s, most researchers and clinicians assumed that these bacteria were harmless contaminants. Few clinicians believed that any form of bacteria could actually survive within the highly acidic environment of the stomach. However, Dr. Barry Marshall, an Australian microbiologist, and Dr. Robin Warren, his pathologist colleague, remained suspicious that *H. pylori* was more than an innocuous contaminant in patients who were diagnosed with peptic ulcers, and so Dr. Marshall subsequently decided to use himself as a guinea pig. After drinking a batch of *H. pylori* bacteria growing in a laboratory culture dish, Dr. Marshall subsequently developed severe gastritis, which was then proven to be caused by the *H. pylori* bacteria that he had ingested. (For their work in demonstrating that *H. pylori* directly caused chronic inflammation of the upper GI tract, Dr. Marshall and Dr. Warren were awarded the 2005 Nobel Prize in Medicine.)

By the end of the 1980s, multiple researchers had determined that chronic infection with *H. pylori* was also a direct cause of stomach (gastric) cancer. A huge prospective public health study, published in the prestigious *New England Journal of Medicine* in 1991, evaluated nearly 139,000 patients within a large health-maintenance organization (HMO). After decades of close follow-up, this clinical research study determined that chronic infection with *H. pylori* was associated with *4 times* the average risk of gastric cancer overall, and a whopping *18-fold increase* in gastric cancer risk in chronically infected women, specifically. African-Americans were also found to be *9 times more likely* to develop stomach cancer if they had a history of *H. pylori* infection [1].

A second potentially malignant condition known to be caused by chronic *H. pylori* infection is "primary gastric lymphoma of mucosa-associated lymphoid tissue," or primary gastric MALT. In fact, this slow-growing form of lymphoma can often be cured simply by eradicating *H. pylori* with antibiotics, although more advanced stages of primary gastric MALT may require chemotherapy, as with other types of lymphoma.

Currently there is some debate regarding the optimal management of chronic *H. pylori* infection, as recent research suggests that *H. pylori* may, ironically, actually *reduce* the risk of cancer of the esophagus. However, most experts currently recommend that *all* confirmed *H. pylori* infections be treated with one of several approved antibiotic regimens.

Human Papilloma Virus (HPV)

HPV is most commonly passed via sexual contact, and oncogenic strains of this virus have long been known to cause more than 95 percent of all cases of cervical cancer in women (as well as genital warts in both men and women). Because this oncogenic virus is known to cause almost all cases of cervical cancer, a great deal of research effort and money have been invested to create HPV vaccines, two of which are currently approved by the Food and Drug Administration in the United States (Gardasil and Cervarix). Gardasil, for which there is the most extensive amount of clinical data, is known to prevent infection with the 4 oncogenic strains of HPV that cause 70 percent of all cervical cancer cases and 90 percent of all cases of genital warts. As these vaccines work by stimulating the immune system to become resistant to HPV infection, they are effective *only* if given *before* the onset of sexual activity (i.e., before any exposure to HPV virus has occurred).

In recent years, there has been growing concern that chronic HPV infection may also be associated with cancers other than cervical cancer. Indeed, there is now substantial clinical and laboratory research data pointing to chronic HPV infection as the primary cause of cancers of the anus, vulva, vagina, penis, and, increasingly, the oropharynx (i.e., the structures within the mouth and throat).

Although HPV vaccines were originally intended for adolescent girls, to prevent cervical cancer, the increasing awareness of other HPV-associated cancers in both men and women has compelled many public health experts to recommend that these very expensive vaccines also be administered to adolescent boys, as well.

Hepatitis B and Hepatitis C Viruses

According to a consensus report issued by the prestigious United States Institute of Medicine in January, 2010, approximately 2 percent of the US population is chronically infected with either the Hepatitis B virus or the Hepatitis C virus. Altogether, *more than 15,000* people die every year in the United States from cirrhosis or liver cancer caused by these oncogenic viruses [2].

Worldwide, Hepatitis B infections account for an estimated 80 percent of all cases of liver cancer. In the United States, and throughout the developed world, the incidence of new Hepatitis B infections has been declining in recent years, following the development of the first effective vaccine against this virus in 1981. In contrast to the declining incidence of Hepatitis B, however, the incidence of Hepatitis C infections continues to rise, as there are currently no effective vaccines available to prevent infection with this oncogenic virus. According to the Centers for Disease Control (United States), today, most people become infected with the Hepatitis C virus by sharing needles or other equipment to inject drugs. (Before 1992, when widespread screening of the blood supply for this virus began in the United States, Hepatitis C was also commonly spread through blood transfusions and organ transplants.) Unprotected sexual contact can also spread the Hepatitis C virus, although the Hepatitis B and HIV viruses are more easily transmitted by unprotected sexual activity. Therefore, the best way to avoid becoming infected with the

Hepatitis C virus, and other dangerous oncogenic viruses, is by avoiding the risky behaviors that can transmit these diseases.

Human Immunodeficiency Virus (HIV/AIDS)

Chronic suppression of the immune system is known to increase the risk of certain cancers, as has been observed in patients who are taking immunosuppressive medications following organ transplantation. Chronic HIV infection also results in varying degrees of immune system suppression. Therefore, it is not surprising that chronic HIV infection is associated with an increased risk of cancer, as well. Two of the three types of cancer most commonly associated with HIV infection are known to be caused by other oncogenic (cancer-causing) viruses. Kaposi's sarcoma is caused by a herpes virus, while cervical cancer, in women, is caused by the human papilloma virus (HPV). The third HIV-associated cancer, non-Hodgkin's lymphoma (NHL), probably arises as a result of mutations in lymphocytes (a type of white blood cell which is part of the immune system) caused directly by the infection of these cells with the HIV virus. Although less common than Kaposi's sarcoma, NHL, and cervical cancer, the risk of other types of cancer is also increased in patients who are infected with the HIV virus, including cancers of the anus, liver, mouth and throat (oropharyngeal carcinoma), lung, testicles, colon, rectum, and skin.

HIV is most commonly transmitted by unprotected sexual activity and intravenous (IV) drug abuse. Therefore, HIV-associated cancers can be prevented, in the vast majority of cases, by abstaining from these high-risk behaviors.

References

1. Parsonnet J, et al. Helicobacter pylori infection and the risk of gastric carcinoma. *New England Journal of Medicine* 1991; 325:1127-1131.

2. "Hepatitis and Liver Cancer: A National Strategy for Prevention and Control of Hepatitis B and C." Institute of Medicine; January 11, 2010.

CHAPTER 10

DIETARY SUPPLEMENTS & CANCER PREVENTION

As I have previously mentioned, there has been an enormous amount of public and scientific interest in dietary supplements as potential cancer prevention agents. The allure of this approach to cancer prevention is understandable, as most dietary supplements, and plant-derived products in particular, tend to be relatively non-toxic, even with relatively large doses. (While it is not always the case that all things natural are safer than synthetic compounds, nonetheless, the safety profile of commonly consumed plant-based supplements is generally very good.) As many health-conscious consumers inherently prefer to use dietary supplements as health adjuncts, it is not surprising that the nutritional supplements industry in the United States, and in other parts of the world, has become an enormous enterprise. Indeed, it has been estimated that the nutritional supplements industry in the United States, alone, generates between $60 billion and $100 billion in sales every year.

Many of us take daily nutritional supplements in an effort to make up for deficiencies in our less-than-healthy modern diets. Many more millions of people also regularly purchase vitamins and other nutritional supplements in the hope that these capsules and tablets might reduce their risk of developing cancer and other serious illnesses. Bombarded by constant advertisements and testimonials about the purported miraculous disease-preventing properties of this vitamin or that supplement, it is easy to get caught up in the hope that a particular vitamin or supplement will significantly reduce one's chances of contracting cancer, or other serious illnesses.

Based upon the biological mechanisms of action for many popular vitamins and nutritional supplements, the enthusiasm for these compounds as potential cancer prevention agents is understandable. However, as recent large, randomized, prospective clinical research trials have begun to supplant older and less reliable dietary survey-based public health studies, the enthusiasm of many cancer researchers has cooled considerably for several micronutrients previously touted as cancer prevention agents, including, in particular, the so-called antioxidant vitamins. Among these formerly promising antioxidant vitamins and nutritional supplements are Vitamin E, Vitamin C, beta-carotene, and selenium. For many years, these supplements were thought by many scientists to have the potential to ward off cancer and cardiovascular disease, the two greatest killers of modern man. However, recent large-scale randomized, placebo-controlled, prospective clinical research trials have found no apparent health benefits associated with the use of these particular vitamin and nutritional supplements; and worse yet, in some cases, the risk of premature death appears to actually be *higher* with the routine use of some of these same antioxidant vitamins and supplements in patients who otherwise eat a balanced diet.

Fortunately, there remains a substantial amount of favorable laboratory and clinical research data available to suggest that other micronutrients may still hold the promise of reducing our risk of cancer and other serious diseases, although almost all scientists and cancer physicians agree that the best source of these potential disease-preventing compounds is in the form of a healthy and balanced diet rich in fresh fruits and colorful vegetables.

Because of the intense interest of both the public and the cancer research community in the use of natural dietary products as part of a comprehensive cancer prevention lifestyle, I will dwell in some detail upon those dietary agents for which there is supportive research data available. As always, I will emphasize prospective randomized clinical research trials whenever they are available and relevant, as these types of research studies provide a much higher level of scientific certainty than the less expensive dietary survey-based clinical studies and laboratory studies that constitute the overwhelming majority of previously published cancer prevention research.

Dietary Flavonoids

Among dietary nutrients that continue to elicit a great deal of interest among cancer prevention researchers are the so-called plant-derived polyphenols. These naturally-occurring compounds have powerful antioxidant effects, as well as multiple other biochemical effects, that appear to inhibit forms of cell damage that have been linked to cancer formation and cancer cell growth.

Moreover, some of these plant-derived compounds may also reduce the risk of cardiovascular disease, as well.

Many of these dietary compounds have been shown to have antitumor activity in cell culture research and animal studies, although these studies often employ much higher doses of these plant-based compounds than can reasonably be ingested and absorbed in a typical human diet. For the most part, the effectiveness of these plant-derived nutrients as cancer prevention agents in humans has not yet been conclusively proven, although there is considerable preclinical research data available to suggest that these compounds are able to interfere with multiple critical biochemical pathways related to cancer cell development and cancer cell growth. These plant-based nutrients are widely found in many types of fruits, vegetables, and legumes, and are also widely available as manufactured dietary supplements.

Flavonoids are polyphenol compounds that occur naturally in plants, including many of the plants that humans consume as food. (There are more than 5,000 known plant flavonoids, and we are just beginning to understand how some of these compounds can potentially enhance our health.) A number of flavonoid compounds have been studied as potential cancer prevention and cancer treatment agents. As with most research looking at natural products as potential disease prevention agents, the cumulative scientific evidence supporting flavonoids as cancer prevention agents has been mixed. However, there is a growing body of research data suggesting a potential role for at least some flavonoids in the prevention of certain types of cancer. Therefore, I will review the most promising flavonoids in this section.

Green Tea Catechins & Related Flavonoids

Catechins are polyphenolic flavonoids that are found in high concentrations in the leaves of the tea plant (*Camelia sinensis*), while non-catechin flavonoids are naturally abdundant in red grapes, red wine, grapefruit, cranberries, strawberries, elderberries, lingonberries, cherry tomatoes, broccoli, olives, shallots, red onions, apples, pears, celery, dark green leafy lettuces, broad beans, and dark chocolate. These flavonoid compounds are potent scavengers of cell-damaging free radicals, and they also appear to interfere with several of the molecular mechanisms whereby cancer cells grow and reproduce.

There is abundant laboratory research suggesting that dietary supplementation with green tea extracts may potentially reduce both the incidence and growth of cancers of the liver, skin, lung, oral cavity, pancreas, bladder, small intestine, colon, prostate, esophagus, and stomach (however, most of the research in this area has been performed in laboratory animals exposed to known carcinogens) [1]. The results of human research with green tea as a potential cancer prevention agent have been more mixed, however (a common dilemma in human disease prevention research, unfortunately). However, at least one human research study, performed in China, found that people who frequently consumed green tea were almost *50 percent less likely* to develop cancers of the stomach and esophagus (both of which are "bad actor" cancers that are rather common in China, and are associated with poor survival rates) [2]. Yet another Chinese study found that drinking two or more cups of green tea a day appeared to reduce the incidence of precancerous changes of the oral cavity [3].

There is emerging clinical data suggesting that green tea catechins, as well as other dietary flavonoids, may also be associated with a decreased risk of colorectal cancer [4, 5, 6]. In a prospective clinical study of nearly 70,000 Chinese women, who were followed for an average of 6 years, regular green tea consumption was associated with a 37 *percent reduction* in the risk of developing colorectal cancer when compared to women who did not regularly drink green tea. An important aspect of this diet survey-based study was that there appeared to be a "dose-response" association between self-reported levels of green tea consumption and colorectal cancer risk. This finding adds greater weight to this survey-based clinical research study's findings that appear to link increased green tea consumption to a decreased risk of colorectal cancer, although other similar epidemiological research studies have failed to identify a link between green tea consumption and colorectal cancer risk [7].

The consumption of both catechin and non-catechin flavonoids may also be associated with a decrease in the risk of other types of cancer, as well. A recently published Italian study evaluated 1,031 patients with ovarian cancer and 2,411 women without ovarian cancer. In this dietary survey-based study, the researchers evaluated dietary flavonoid intake among these two large groups of women. After adjusting for other known ovarian cancer risk factors present in these women volunteers, the researchers determined that the increased consumption of flavonol-rich fruits and vegetables appeared to be associated with a *nearly 40 percent reduction* in the risk of developing ovarian cancer, while a diet rich in tea-derived catechins and isoflavones from soy foods appeared to reduce the risk of ovarian cancer by *nearly 50 percent.*

Because diet survey-based studies, such as this Italian study, provide relatively low levels of clinical research evidence, this study's finding of a very significant reduction in ovarian cancer risk among women who regularly consumed large amounts of dietary flavonols and isoflavones certainly warrants further study in randomized, prospective, placebo-controlled, blinded clinical research trials [8]. Similarly, a prospective Swedish dietary survey-based study involving 61,507 women, and with an average follow-up of more than 15 years, demonstrated a significant reduction in the risk of ovarian cancer associated with regular consumption of both green tea and black tea. Importantly, these researchers also identified an apparent dose-dependent relationship, whereby increasing levels of tea intake appeared to be associated with a progressively decreasing incidence of ovarian cancer. Indeed, the consumption of 2 or more cups of tea per day appeared to be associated with a *nearly 50 percent reduction* in the risk of developing ovarian cancer when compared to seldom or never drinking tea [9].

As with virtually all cancer prevention studies, the clinical data on tea-derived catechins, as well as other dietary flavonoids, is mixed. For every study showing an apparent cancer reduction benefit associated with catechins and other flavonoids, there is a study showing no apparent reduction in the risk of cancer. However, given the lack of significant toxicity associated with reasonable levels of green tea intake (and other plant-based flavonoids, as well), these naturally-occurring dietary compounds should be considered as components of a cancer prevention lifestyle.

Proanthocyanidins

Proanthocyanidins are widely found in fruits, vegetables, seeds, flowers, nuts, and pine tree bark. These flavonoids are especially common in cranberries, black currants, green tea, and black tea. Grape seeds are also a particularly rich source of proanthocyanidins. Chemically, proanthocyanidins are composed of chains of the same catechin molecules that are thought to give green tea its putative anti-cancer properties.

While there is only very limited and preliminary human data available regarding proanthocyanidins and cancer prevention, there is a considerable amount of available laboratory research data on proanthocyanidins using cancer cell cultures and laboratory mice. These preclinical studies have shown potential anti-cancer activity by proanthocyanidins against cancers of the skin, brain, lung, breast, prostate, stomach, and colon [10, 11].

Isoflavones

Isoflavones, yet another member of the huge plant-based flavonoid group, are most abundantly found in soybean-derived foods, including tofu. Unlike resveratrol, green tea catechins, and curcumin, soy-derived isoflavones are highly bioavailable, and are readily absorbed by the GI tract.

As with many other plant-derived polyphenols, soy isoflavones act as a weak form of estrogen in humans, and this has led to considerable concern regarding the potential of these nutrients to stimulate the growth of new breast cancers, or to spur cancer recurrence in breast cancer survivors. Indeed, estrogen-sensitive breast cancer cells growing in culture dishes are stimulated to divide when low concentrations of soy isoflavones are added, although higher concentrations of genistein, the primary isoflavone found in soy foods, actually appear to block estrogen hormone receptors on human breast cancer cells, and reduce breast cancer cell growth. Not surprisingly, the clinical research data in humans regarding isoflavones and breast cancer prevention has been mixed, to date. However, there are multiple recent prospective public health studies that have associated increased soy isoflavone intake with a *reduced* risk of breast cancer, particularly when soy-based foods are consumed around the time of adolescence and early adulthood (i.e., when the female breast is undergoing its most rapid phase of development) [12, 13].

There is also public health research data available suggesting that increased soy intake might also reduce the risk of developing colorectal adenomas, which are the premalignant polyps that give rise to the vast majority of colorectal cancers. Curiously, however, some studies suggest that *women* may derive more benefit from soy isoflavone intake than *men* with respect to colorectal adenoma prevention [14]. Other recently published public health research data also suggests that high levels of soy isoflavone intake may be associated with a decreased risk of developing colorectal cancer, as well [15].

As I have noted in a previous section, soy isoflavones may also decrease the risk of ovarian cancer. I will also further discuss the role of isoflavones in the prevention of breast cancer and prostate cancer later in this book.

Quercetin

Quercetin is a plant flavonoid that is naturally found in capers, apples, green tea, red onions, red grapes, tomatoes, citrus fruits, broccoli, leafy green vegetables, cherries, raspberries, lingonberries, and cranberries. Recent animal studies have produced contradictory results regarding quercetin's potential effectiveness as a cancer prevention nutrient.

There is, however, both laboratory and clinical (human) research data suggesting that quercetin, in addition to other dietary flavonoids, may have potential anti-cancer effects against colorectal cancer and pancreatic cancer [16, 17].

Tannins

Naturally occurring sources of tannins include red wine, green tea, pomegranate juice, persimmons, strawberries, blueberries, cranberries, walnuts, pecans, hazelnuts, and beers that are brewed with large amounts of hops.

Pomegranate juice, which is rich in both tannins and phenolic acids, has recently been studied as a potential cancer prevention agent, and as a prostate cancer prevention agent in particular (and which I will discuss later in the expanded chapter on prostate cancer). One recently published laboratory research study has also found that treating aggressive human breast cancer cells with pomegranate juice extract dramatically reduced the ability of these cancer cells to migrate and invade [18].

Non-Flavonoid Plant-Based Nutrients

In addition to flavonoids, many other plant-based compounds hold promise as potential cancer prevention agents. In this section, I will discuss non-flavonoid natural compounds for which there is at least a reasonable body of supportive research data.

Resveratrol

Resveratrol, which belongs to the class of plant-derived chemicals (phytochemicals) known as non-flavonoid polyphenols, has recently attracted the attention of scientists specializing in cancer, cardiovascular disease, and longevity research. Naturally-occurring sources of resveratrol include red and purple grapes, red wine, dark red and dark blue berries, and peanuts.

The available research data on resveratrol's anti-cancer properties has, in general, shown that this polyphenolic compound can impair the growth of a variety of different human cancer cells growing in laboratory cell cultures, including breast, prostate, stomach, colon, pancreas, and thyroid cancer cells [19]. When tested in laboratory animals exposed to known carcinogens, resveratrol supplements have been shown to reduce the risk of several types of cancers, including cancers of the colon, rectum, esophagus, and breast [20, 21]. Other studies of resveratrol suggest the possibility that this intriguing molecule may also reduce the risk of cardiovascular disease, and may also increase the activity of genes associated with a prolonged lifespan (at least in laboratory animals).

One apparent limitation of resveratrol is that it must be consumed frequently, and in higher doses, in order to significantly increase the level of resveratrol in the blood and other tissues (resveratrol is not readily absorbed, and once it is absorbed, it is rapidly metabolized in the body).

As with several other polyphenolic compounds, resveratrol does exhibit some weak estrogen-like properties, and so women with a history of estrogen dependent cancers, including cancers of the breast, ovary, and uterus, should be aware that, at least theoretically, large doses of resveratrol could potentially stimulate the growth of breast cancer and other estrogen-dependent types of cancer.

While it is not currently known if oral supplementation with resveratrol can significantly reduce the risk of cancer in humans, several prospective randomized, placebo-controlled clinical resveratrol research trials are already underway at this time.

Sulforaphane

Sulforaphane has stimulated a great deal of interest among cancer prevention scientists, recently. Sulforaphane belongs to a group of compounds known as isothiocyanates, and is most abundant in young broccoli sprouts and other cruciferous (brassica) vegetables, including mature broccoli, brussels sprouts, broccoli raab, cabbage, bok choy, chinese broccoli, kale, collard greens, mustard greens, turnip greens, cauliflower, kohlrabi, radishes, arugula, and watercress.

Sulforaphane has been shown to inhibit the development of certain cancers, and to increase cancer cell death, in cultured cancer cells as well as in mice transplanted with human cancer cells. To date, sulforaphane has shown anti-cancer activity, via multiple biochemical pathways, against cancers of the breast, prostate, lung, pancreas, oral cavity, colon, and rectum [22, 23].

Other epidemiological studies have suggested that a diet rich in cruciferous vegetables may also reduce the risk of non-Hodgkin's lymphoma [24, 25].

An area of particular interest to me is the prevention of pancreas cancer, which remains a highly lethal form of cancer. Unfortunately, this type of cancer remains highly resistant to cure by surgery, chemotherapy, or radiation therapy. Therefore, the prevention of pancreas cancer, whenever possible, offers a much greater hope of decreasing the death rate due to this aggressive form of cancer than any currently available treatment.

Recently published laboratory research studies suggest that sulforaphane may be significantly toxic against human pancreas cancer cells. In one of these studies, human pancreatic cancer cells were injected into mice with deficient immune systems. Daily sulforaphane injections, over a period of 3 weeks, reduced the size of the resulting pancreatic cancer tumors by an average of 40 percent when compared with tumor-implanted mice that received only placebo injections. Thus, this study suggests that sulforaphane may not only potentially reduce the risk of pancreatic cancer, but may also offer another possible mode of treatment in patients who have already developed this highly aggressive form of cancer [26, 27].

(I will discuss the potential role of sulforaphane in the prevention of breast cancer in the expanded chapter on breast cancer, later in this book.)

Curcumin

Curcumin is a non-flavonoid polyphenol that is found in turmeric, the primary spice used to make curry. Curcumin has long been advocated as a cancer prevention agent. As with green tea catechins, curcumin is not readily absorbed following oral ingestion. Also, as is common in cancer prevention research, the observed effects of curcumin on cancer risk have been rather variable between different research studies. However, in my view, there is enough favorable research data to suggest that curcumin is likely to have potentially significant effects against specific types of cancer.

Based upon research using laboratory mice, large oral doses of curcumin appear to significantly reduce the incidence of both precancerous colon adenomas and colon cancer tumors [28-30].

In yet another animal model of colorectal cancer, laboratory rats that were fed either curcumin or green tea supplements were much less likely to develop colorectal cancer than rats that did not receive either of these dietary supplements. This colorectal cancer prevention effect was especially potent in rats that received *both* curcumin and green tea catechin supplements, which appeared to significantly reduce the incidence of colorectal cancer (i.e., when compared to the animals that did not receive either supplement) [31].

In another intriguing laboratory research study, human pancreatic cancer tumors were established in immune-deficient mice, and the animals were then divided into 3 treatment groups consisting of omega-3 fatty acid (fish oil) supplements, curcumin supplements, and a combination of omega-3 fatty acid and curcumin supplements. Although responses in laboratory mice often do not predict responses in humans, the findings of this research study were nonetheless rather spectacular, given the high degree of resistance of pancreatic cancer to currently available therapies. The mice that received fish oil supplements experienced a 25 percent reduction in the size of their tumors (when compared to the control group mice that were fed corn oil supplements), while the mice that were fed curcumin supplements experienced a 43 percent reduction in the size of their implanted human pancreatic cancer tumors. Moreover, the mice who received *both* omega-3 fatty acid *and* curcumin supplements experienced a dramatic *72 percent reduction in the size* of their pancreatic cancer tumors, suggesting a potent additive effect between omega-3 fatty acids and curcumin against human pancreatic cancer tumors [32]. (Once again, whether or not these findings are reproducible in humans with pancreatic cancer is unknown at this time.)

Another recent laboratory study suggests that the combination of curcumin with other natural dietary compounds might also synergistically act to reduce the risk of pancreatic cancer, and to shrink existing pancreatic cancer tumors. In this study, cultured human pancreatic cancer cells were treated with soy-based isoflavones and curcumin, both separately and in combination. While both soy isoflavones and curcumin, when administered individually, inhibited pancreas cancer cell growth, and induced cancer cell death, the combination of the two dietary compounds resulted in a significantly greater effect than when each was given alone. The results of this study, therefore, suggest a potential role for the combination of soy isoflavones and curcumin in the prevention and treatment of pancreatic cancer [33]. (Once again, whether these laboratory observations will hold up in humans remains to be seen, but the biochemical mechanisms whereby these dietary agents impair pancreatic cell growth and survival have been worked out, and suggest that these dietary compounds may indeed be active in tumors growing in humans.)

Other laboratory studies have evaluated curcumin's effects on human cancer cells growing in culture, and have demonstrated that curcumin is capable of blocking key metabolic pathways in leukemia and lymphoma cells, as well as in multiple types of gastrointestinal cancers, urinary tract cancers, breast cancer, ovarian cancer, head and neck cancer, lung cancer, melanoma, brain cancer, and sarcomas [34].

While there is a growing abundance of laboratory research data regarding potential anti-cancer effects associated with curcumin, there is still very little human clinical data available. However, an early-phase prospective clinical trial of curcumin from the M.D. Anderson Cancer Center has recently reported its findings. In this study, 21 patients with advanced pancreatic cancer received daily oral curcumin supplements, and these patients were then reassessed every 2 months. In addition to radiographic imaging studies of their tumors, pancreatic cancer tumor markers were measured in the blood of these patients every 2 months. In one patient who received curcumin, no tumor growth or spread was noted for more than 18 months, which is remarkable for advanced pancreatic cancer. In a second patient, curcumin supplementation was associated with a 73% reduction in tumor size, which is also a dramatic response for pancreatic cancer (though the tumor response in this patient turned out to be temporary in nature). Although the tumors of the remaining 19 patients did not appear to respond as dramatically, as occurred with the first two patients, decreased levels of pancreatic cancer tumor markers in the blood of these remaining patients suggested that the tumors of these patients were also responding to the curcumin supplements [35]. Why only two patients' tumors clinically responded, however transiently, so dramatically to curcumin and the others did not is unclear at this time. However, all patients who received curcumin showed at least "biochemical evidence" of anti-cancer activity in their blood. Although the overall clinical effects of curcumin in this early-phase clinical research study were not very dramatic in absolute terms, the fact that *any* of the patients with advanced pancreatic cancer in this study experienced any clinically detectable benefit from this dietary supplement is actually quite remarkable. Advanced pancreatic cancers, such as these, are refractory to all currently approved treatments, and so even incremental clinical signs of treatment response, such as were demonstrated in this study, are a cause for hope. (Based upon the results of this small early-phase clinical study, additional and larger prospective clinical pancreatic cancer research trials with curcumin are certainly warranted and, indeed, 3 such studies are currently underway at this time.)

In some studies, curcumin has been associated with toxic effects at higher doses, and may even *increase* the risk of tumor formation under some conditions [36]. Because of these potential adverse effects, it is unclear, at this time, whether or not curcumin should be routinely used as a cancer prevention agent. However, curcumin should certainly be further studied as a potential cancer prevention agent through well-controlled prospective, randomized human clinical trials. Additionally, curcumin may hold promise for patients with pancreatic cancer, particularly in view of this cancer's dismal prognosis, and its high degree of resistance to current therapies.

Lupeol

Lupeol has only recently come to the attention of cancer preventions research scientists and, therefore, the amount of research data available at this time is limited. Lupeol is naturally abundant in mangoes, and is also found in strawberries, red grapes, figs, olives, tomatoes, peppers, and cucumbers. In addition to its anti-inflammatory properties, lupeol has been shown, in laboratory research, to inhibit several different biological pathways necessary for cancer cell growth and survival. In laboratory testing, lupeol has shown significant activity, specifically, against cancers of the head and neck, skin, prostate, and pancreas.

At this time, there is no human research data available on lupeol as a cancer prevention agent. However, as with curcumin, there is some highly intriguing laboratory data suggesting that lupeol may inhibit the growth and survival of human pancreas cancer cells and other highly aggressive types of cancer.

In one important study, human pancreatic cancer cells growing in culture were exposed to increasing concentrations of lupeol, with a resulting dose-dependent decrease in cancer cell growth, and an increase in cancer cell death. Lupeol treatment was also found to significantly reduce levels of the cancer-associated protein Ras, which is commonly mutated in pancreas cancer, and in other aggressive forms of cancer [37].

Another similar study looked at the effects of lupeol on chemotherapy-resistant human pancreatic cancer cells growing in culture, and on tumors created from the same cancer cells after they were transplanted into mice with deficient immune systems. Lupeol treatment significantly reduced the growth of these highly resistant and highly aggressive human pancreatic cancer cells growing in culture, and significantly reduced the growth of the implanted tumors growing in laboratory mice. Therefore, as with curcumin, lupeol appears to have potential activity against aggressive pancreatic cancer cells [38].

In addition to activity against pancreas cancer cells, lupeol has also been shown to inhibit the growth of another highly aggressive cancer, metastatic melanoma. In at least one study, lupeol inhibited the growth of metastatic human melanoma cancer cells growing in culture, but did not inhibit the growth of normal human skin pigment cells (melanocytes), from which melanoma arises. As with many of the other dietary compounds that have been studied as potential cancer prevention agents, lupeol was shown to directly interfere with multiple specific, critical biological pathways in cultured human melanoma cells. In the second part of this research study, these same aggressive melanoma cancer cells were then injected into mice with defective immune systems. Treatment of these mice with lupeol resulted in decreased growth of the implanted melanoma tumors when compared to mice that did not receive lupeol. Thus, as with highly aggressive and treatment-resistant pancreatic cancer cells, similarly aggressive and treatment-resistant metastatic melanoma cancer cells also appear to be inhibited by lupeol, at least under laboratory conditions [39].

Prostate cancer cells may also be susceptible to inhibition by lupeol. In one laboratory study, lupeol was found to directly inhibit multiple specific biological pathways related to prostate cancer cell growth and survival [40].

Phytosterols

Phytosterols are plant-based compounds that are chemically similar to cholesterol (which is found only in animals). As is the case with many of the other plant-based nutrients that I have discussed thus far, phytosterols are poorly absorbed from the GI tract. Moreover, once absorbed, phytosterols are rapidly excreted into the bile by the liver, and eliminated from the body.

Phytosterols are known to reduce the concentration of LDL (the "bad cholesterol") in the blood. While there is very little human data available regarding potential anti-cancer properties associated with phytosterols, there is an increasing amount of laboratory data available. These laboratory studies have identified an apparent inhibitory effect of dietary phytosterols on cancers of the lung, stomach, colon, ovary, prostate, and breast [41, 42].

Thus, based upon laboratory research, at least, phytosterols may have a potentially important role to play not only in the reduction of cardiovascular disease, but, perhaps, as cancer prevention agents, as well.

Flaxseed & Omega-3 Fatty Acids

Flaxseed oil contains two types of compounds that may have anti-cancer activity, lignans and omega-3 fatty acids. Similar to soy-derived isoflavones, flaxseed lignans are known to act as phytoestrogens (plant-based compounds that weakly reproduce the effects of estrogen, the primary sex hormone in females). Omega-3 fatty acids, which are abundant in flaxseed (as well as in fish, canola oil, and walnuts), are known to reduce inflammation in the body, and may potentially reduce the risk of both cardiovascular disease and cancer.

Recent cancer prevention studies of omega-3 fatty acids have determined that multiple important cancer growth and survival biochemical pathways are significantly inhibited by omega-3 fatty acids [43].

Fish oils, which are rich in omega-3 fatty acids (as with flaxseed, canola oil, and walnuts), have been intensively studied as potential disease-prevention agents. Multiple laboratory and clinical research studies have shown that omega-3 fatty acids have numerous beneficial health effects, including potent anti-inflammatory effects. Most of the research on omega-3 fatty acids has been dedicated to their cardiovascular protective effects, and their ability to reduce the risk of coronary artery disease and peripheral vascular disease. Increasingly, however, newer omega-3 fatty acid research studies are suggesting that these dietary oils may also have important cancer prevention properties as well (and in particular, against cancers of the colon, breast, pancreas, and prostate) [44].

As I have mentioned previously, however, just because a supplement is "natural" does not mean that it is non-toxic. Excessive fish oil intake can expose patients to elevated levels of mercury and other heavy metals. Additionally, high levels of omega-3 fatty acids can also thin the blood to the point where excessive bleeding can occur with minor injuries or surgical procedures. Finally, increased intake of omega-3 fatty acids can be toxic to some patients with underlying kidney disease. Therefore, I always recommend that patients check with their primary physician before initiating new dietary supplements of any kind.

Vitamins

The last 10 years have been rather unkind to vitamins in terms of their potential as cancer prevention agents. As much of the data on nutritional and dietary supplements that I have thus far presented reveals, most disease prevention research has been performed using lower-level research methodologies, including epidemiological (public health) research based primarily upon surveys, and laboratory studies consisting of experiments using cell cultures and laboratory animals. Unfortunately, the findings of most low-level studies, such as these, are rarely validated in prospective, randomized human research trials. When randomized, placebo-controlled, blinded clinical research trials have been performed, most vitamins have been found to be ineffective as cancer prevention agents, and some of these same vitamins have even been found to be potentially harmful. This has particularly been the case with the so-called antioxidant vitamins.

Antioxidant Vitamins (Vitamin C, Vitamin E, Beta-Carotene)

Over the past 10 years, multiple large prospective, randomized, controlled human clinical research studies have been performed to evaluate antioxidant vitamins that have, for years, been widely recommended, and utilized, as cancer prevention agents. Herein lies an important lesson for all of us, because Vitamin C, Vitamin E, and several members of the Vitamin A family, had all previously been extensively studied through epidemiological survey-based methods, as well as in the laboratory. Based upon our current understanding of the mechanisms of cancer cell development, growth, and spread, as well as our understanding of the mechanisms of action of these antioxidant vitamins, large doses of these vitamins were *supposed to work* by sopping up DNA-damaging free radicals that are constantly being generated as products of cellular metabolism. Numerous low-level research studies of antioxidant vitamins had raised hopes that these potent free radical scavengers would protect our cells from genetic damage and could, therefore, reduce the risk of cancer-causing DNA mutations. Instead, when "gold standard" rigorous prospective clinical research studies were finally performed with these vitamins, the results were extremely disappointing, to say the least.

Multiple large-scale prospective, randomized, placebo-controlled clinical research trials over the past decade have shown that Vitamin E supplements do *not* appear to reduce the risk of cancer. Moreover, there have been recent large-scale prospective clinical trials that have identified a potential *increase* in the overall risk of death among study volunteers who were secretly randomized to receive Vitamin E supplements. Similarly, other prospective, randomized clinical studies involving tens of thousands of volunteers have evaluated the impact of beta-carotene (a member of the Vitamin A family) in preventing lung cancer and other cancers. Not only did these studies find no apparent cancer prevention benefit associated with beta-carotene, but they also identified an *increased* risk of lung cancer among smokers who were secretly randomized to receive beta-carotene [45-49].

A comprehensive meta-analysis of 67 different prospective, randomized clinical research trials of the most commonly taken antioxidant supplements (e.g., beta-carotene, Vitamin A, Vitamin C, Vitamin E, and selenium) was performed by the much-respected Cochrane Database of Systematic Reviews in 2008. Altogether, these 67 clinical trials included more than 232,000 patient volunteers. This massive meta-analysis study determined that Vitamin A supplements were associated with a *16 percent increase* in the relative risk of death (mortality) due to any cause, while beta-carotene and Vitamin E supplements were associated with a *7 percent and 4 percent increase* in all-cause mortality, respectively. Selenium and Vitamin C supplementation, on the other hand, did not appear to be associated with any increase *or* decrease in mortality [50].

Yet another huge meta-analysis studied 14 prospectively conducted clinical trials that, together, included more than 170,000 patient volunteers. These clinical trials studied the effects of the antioxidant supplements beta-carotene, Vitamin A, Vitamin C, Vitamin E, and selenium on the risk of cancers of the esophagus, stomach, colon, rectum, pancreas, and liver. This huge meta-analysis study failed to find any impact on the incidence of these highly lethal cancers following supplementation with these antioxidant dietary supplements. Moreover, once again, regularly taking supplements of either Vitamin E or beta-carotene, or both, appeared to *increase* the risk of death [51].

Therefore, while some diehard fans of antioxidant vitamins and supplements continue to argue that these enormous prospective, randomized, placebo-controlled clinical trials are poorly designed, or that the chemical form or dose of antioxidants utilized are flawed, there is now a massive amount of very high-level clinical research data that, repeatedly, appears to show no cancer risk-reduction properties associated with supplements of beta-carotene, Vitamin A, Vitamin C, Vitamin E, or selenium. In fact, there is a growing body of high-level clinical research data suggesting that taking routine supplements of beta-carotene or Vitamin E may actually *increase* the overall risk of death.

Lycopene

Lycopene is closely related, chemically, to the Vitamin A family, although it does not perform any of the biochemical functions associated with Vitamin A. Lycopene, like other so-called carotenoids, is a potent antioxidant, and is able to detoxify cell-damaging free radicals. Lycopene is abundant in many red and orange fruits and vegetables, including tomatoes, carrots, watermelon, red bell peppers, pink guava, pink grapefruit, papaya, and rosehips. Cooked byproducts of tomatoes are especially rich in absorbable lycopene, including tomato juice, tomato paste, tomato sauce, and tomato ketchup.

Most of the interest in lycopene as a potential cancer prevention agent has been directed towards prostate cancer, based upon the results of previous low-level laboratory and public health studies. Although recent prospective human research data suggests that increased lycopene intake may indeed be associated with a decreased overall risk of cancer, ironically, it now appears highly questionable that lycopene reduces prostate cancer risk. For example, a recent prospective clinical study of 997 middle-aged men, with an average follow-up of nearly 13 years, evaluated the levels of lycopene in their blood versus the incidence of cancer in this group of patient volunteers. While higher levels of lycopene in the blood appeared to be associated with a *57 percent decrease* in the *relative* overall risk of cancer, high levels of lycopene did *not* appear to offer any protection against prostate cancer [52].

Folate, Vitamin B6 and Vitamin B12

As with the antioxidant vitamins, recent prospective, randomized, double-blind, placebo-controlled clinical research trials have shown no apparent cancer prevention effects associated with folate, Vitamin B6, or Vitamin B12 supplements. In fact, one recent such study, which followed nearly 7,000 patient volunteers for an average of more than 6 years, actually identified an *increased* risk of cancer, and cancer-related death, associated with folate, Vitamin B6, and Vitamin B12 supplements [53].

Vitamin D

Despite the dismal recent news regarding the common antioxidant vitamins (and selenium), there is still actually some reason for hope that at least one vitamin, Vitamin D, may possess the ability to reduce cancer risk. (Interestingly, Vitamin D functions more like a hormone than a vitamin.)

Vitamin D primarily regulates the level of calcium in our bodies, but is thought to have other important biological effects as well. (One very important additional function of Vitamin D is its ability to stimulate the immune system, which may account for its ability to inhibit the growth of multiple different types of human cancers.)

In healthy individuals, most of the Vitamin D in our bodies is created as a result of skin exposure to sunlight. In areas where sunlight is not abundant, and in people with darker skin pigmentation (and in the elderly), Vitamin D deficiency is very common. These clinical observations have spurred research into the relationship between sunlight levels and cancer incidence, with the resulting finding that people who live in areas of the world with low-levels of sunlight are *more likely* to develop certain types of cancers, including cancers of the colon, rectum, breast, ovary and prostate. This frequently observed "North-South" variation in cancer incidence has given rise to the hypothesis that decreased Vitamin D levels in the body may be associated with an increased risk of certain types of cancer. Moreover, there is additional epidemiological research available to suggest that Vitamin D, when taken as a supplement, may reduce the risk of cancers of the breast, colon, prostate, ovary, lungs, and pancreas [54].

The strongest evidence in support of Vitamin D as a cancer prevention agent is in the area of colorectal cancer prevention. A Harvard University study, published in 2008, analyzed 17 previous epidemiological Vitamin D research studies. The incidence of colorectal adenomas, which are the polyps that give rise to nearly all colorectal cancers, was *reduced by 30 percent* in patients with high levels of Vitamin D in their blood [55]. Epidemiological studies from Japan have also shown a similar, and significant, degree of decreased colorectal cancer risk associated with increasing intake of Vitamin D (and calcium), and with increased levels of Vitamin D in the blood [56, 57].

As with all areas of medical research, and in disease prevention studies in particular, it is easy to find contradictory data. Indeed, the large prospective, randomized, placebo-controlled Women's Health Initiative study, which included more than 36,000 postmenopausal women, found *no decrease* in the risk of colorectal cancer associated with the intake of calcium and Vitamin D supplements. However, critics of this study point out that the daily Vitamin D supplement of 400 International Units (IU) per day used in this study is considerably below the 1,000 to 2,000 IU daily dose that has been reported to decrease colorectal cancer risk in other studies [58]. (For example, a large meta-analysis of previously published Vitamin D studies found that daily doses of Vitamin D of 1,000 IU per day were associated with a *nearly 50 percent reduction* in the incidence of colorectal cancer [59]).

There is considerable additional research data suggesting that higher levels of Vitamin D in the blood may reduce the risk of breast cancer. For example, in one case-control study, blood levels of Vitamin D were measured in more than 1,000 breast cancer patients, and in more than 1,000 age-matched control patients without breast cancer. Blood levels of Vitamin D above 40 nanograms per milliliter (ng/ml) were associated with a *44 percent observed decrease* in the risk of breast cancer (and a *54 percent decrease* in breast cancer risk among postmenopausal women, specifically) when compared with the women who had decreased levels of Vitamin D in their blood [60]. Similarly, a meta-analysis of 26 previously published Vitamin D studies found that high levels of Vitamin D in the blood were associated with a *45 percent reduction* in the incidence of breast cancer. Higher blood levels of calcium were also associated with a *19 percent reduction* in the risk of breast cancer [61]. Finally, yet a third case-control breast cancer study that evaluated Vitamin D levels also indentified a remarkably similar *48 percent decrease* in the risk of breast cancer associated with higher Vitamin D levels in the blood [62].

Although the data tends not to be as strong as it is for colorectal cancer, there is intriguing evidence that Vitamin D may have anti-cancer effects against prostate cancer, as well. In a small pilot study, 15 patients with recurrence of their prostate cancer were given 2,000 IU of Vitamin D per day. In 9 of these patients with treatment-refractory prostate cancer, the prostate cancer marker PSA either declined, or remained stable for as long as 21 months, suggesting a clinically significant anti-cancer effect by Vitamin D. Moreover, the time required for PSA levels in the blood to double in value was increased in 14 of these 15 patients after Vitamin D supplements were initiated [63].

Vitamin D, among all known vitamins, appears to have the greatest likelihood of truly functioning as a cancer prevention agent. While various studies have suggested that Vitamin D may reduce the risk of as many as 17 different types of cancer, the available laboratory and clinical data most strongly support an anti-cancer effect for this vitamin against colorectal cancer, breast cancer, and prostate cancer. However, not everyone should take large doses of Vitamin D, as the unmonitored use of this potent hormone-like vitamin can cause dangerous elevations in the level of calcium in the blood, as well as calcifications in the soft tissues of the body, kidney failure, pancreatitis, and gastrointestinal ulcers. However, in healthy patients, 1,000 to 2,000 IU of Vitamin D per day is generally well-tolerated. (Prior to starting Vitamin D supplements, you should certainly discuss the risks and benefits of high-dose Vitamin D supplementation with your physician.)

References

1. Lambert JD, et al. Inhibition of carcinogenesis by polyphenols: evidence from laboratory investigations. *American Journal of Clinical Nutrition* 2005; 81:284S-291S.

2. Sun CL, Yuan JM, Lee MJ, Yang CS, Gao YT, Ross RK, Yu MC. Urinary tea polyphenols in relation to gastric and esophageal cancers: A prospective study of men in Shanghai, China. *Carcinoma* 2002; 23(9):1497–1503.

3. Dufresne CJ, Farnworth ER. A review of latest research findings on the health promotion properties of tea. *Journal of Nutritional Biochemistry* 2001; 12:404–421.

4. Kyle JA, et al. Dietary flavonoid intake and colorectal cancer: a case control study. *British Journal of Nutrition* 2009; 7:1-8.

5. Theodoratou E, et al. Dietary flavonoids and the risk of colorectal cancer. *Cancer Epidemiology, Biomarkers & Prevention* 2007; 16:684-693.

6. Bobe G. et al. Dietary flavonoids and colorectal adenoma recurrence in the Polyp Prevention Trial. *Cancer, Epidemiology & Prevention* 2008; 17:1344-1353.

7. Yang G, et al. Prospective cohort study of green tea consumption and colorectal cancer risk in women. *Cancer Epidemiology, Biomarkers & Prevention* 2007; 16:1219-1223.

8. Rossi M, et al. Flavonoids and ovarian cancer risk: A case-control study in Italy. *International Journal of Cancer* 2008; 123:895-898.

9. Larsson SC & Wolk A. Tea consumption and ovarian cancer risk in a population-based cohort. *Archives of Internal Medicine* 2005; 165:2683-2686.

10. Neto C. Cranberry and its phytochemicals: a review of in vitro anticancer studies. *Journal of Nutrition* 2007; 137:186S-193S.

11. Ferguson PJ, et al. In vivo inhibition of growth of human tumor lines by flavonoid fractions from cranberry extract. *Nutrition & Cancer* 2006; 56:86-94.

12. Iwasaki M, et al. Dietary isoflavone intake and breast cancer risk in case-control studies in Japanese, Japanese Brazilians, and non-Japanese Brazilians. *Breast Cancer Research & Treatment* 2009; 116:401-411.

13. Lee SA, et al. Adolescent and adult soy food intake and breast cancer risk: results from the Shanghai Women's Health Study. *American Journal of Clinical Nutrition* 2009; 89:1920-1926.

14. Akhter M, et al. Dietary isoflavone and the risk of colorectal adenoma: a case-control study in Japan. *British Journal of Cancer* 2009; 100:1812-1816.

15. Yang G, et al. Prospective cohort study of soy food intake and colorectal cancer risk in women. *American Journal of Clinical Nutrition* 2009; 89:577-583.

16. Kyle JA, et al. Dietary flavonoid intake and colorectal cancer: a case control study. *British Journal of Nutrition* 2009; 2009 Sep 7:1-8. [Epub ahead of print].

17. Lambert JD, et al. Inhibition of carcinogenesis by polyphenols: evidence from laboratory investigations. *American Journal of Clinical Nutrition* 2005; 81:284S-291S.

18. Khan GN, et al. Pomegranate fruit extract impairs invasion and motility in human breast cancer. *Integrative Cancer Therapy* 2009; 8:242-253.

19. Aggarwal BB, et al. Role of resveratrol in prevention and therapy of cancer: preclinical and clinical studies. *Anticancer Research* 2004; 24:2783-2840.

20. Bhat KP, et al. Estrogenic and antiestrogenic properties of resveratrol in mammary tumor models. *Cancer Research* 2001; 61:7456-7463.

21. Banerjee S, et al. Suppression of 7,12-dimethylbenz(a)anthracene-induced mammary carcinogenesis in rats by resveratrol: role of nuclear factor-kappaB, cyclooxygenase 2, and matrix metalloprotease 9. *Cancer Research* 2002; 62:4945-4954.

22. Clarke JD, et al. Multi-targeted prevention of cancer by sulforaphane. *Cancer Letters* 2008; 269:291-304.

23. Juge N, et al. Molecular basis for chemoprevention by sulforaphane: a comprehensive review. *Cell & Molecular Life Sciences* 2007; 64:1105-1127.

24. Zhang SM, et al. Intakes of fruits, vegetables, and related nutrients and the risk of non-Hodgkin's lymphoma among women. *Cancer, Epidemiology, Biomarkers & Prevention* 2000; 9:477-485.

25. Michaud DS, et al. Fruit and vegetable intake and incidence of bladder cancer in a male prospective cohort. *Journal of the National Cancer Institute* 1999; 91:605-613.

26. Pham NA, et al. The dietary isothiocyanate sulforaphane targets pathways of apoptosis, cell cycle arrest, and oxidative stress in human pancreatic cancer cells and inhibits tumor growth in severe combined immunodeficient mice. *Molecular Cancer Therapeutics* 2004; 3:1239-1248.

27. Kallifatidis G, et al. Sulforaphane targets pancreatic tumor-initiating cells by NF-kappa B-induced antiapoptotic signaling. *Gut* 2009; 58:949-963.

28. Huang MT, et al. Inhibitory effects of dietary curcumin on forestomach, duodenal, and colon carcinogenesis in mice. *Cancer Research* 1994; 54:5841–5847.

29. Perkins S, et al. Chemopreventive efficacy and pharmacokinetics of curcumin in the min/+ mouse, a model of familial adenomatous polyposis. *Cancer Epidemiology, Biomarkers & Prevention* 2002; 11:535–540.

30. Johnson JJ, Mukhtar H. Curcumin for chemoprevention of colon cancer. *Cancer Letters* 2007; 255:170-181.

31. Xu G, et al. Combination of curcumin and green tea catechins prevents dimethylhydrazine-induced colon carcinogenesis. *Food & Chemical Toxicology* 2009; Oct 25, [Epub ahead of print].

32. Swamy MV, et al. Prevention and treatment of pancreatic cancer by curcumin in combination with omega-3 fatty acids. *Nutrition and Cancer* 2008; 60:81-89.

33. Wang Z, et al. Synergistic effects of multiple natural products in pancreatic cancer cells. *Life Sciences* 2008; 83:293-300.

34. Anand P, et al. Curcumin and cancer: an "old-age" disease with an "age-old" solution. *Cancer Letters* 2008; 267:133-163.

35. Dhillon N, et al. Phase II trial of curcumin in patients with advanced pancreatic cancer. *Clinical Cancer Research* 2008; 14:4491-4499.

36. Lopez-Lazaro M. Anticancer and carcinogenic properties of curcumin: considerations for its clinical development as a cancer chemopreventive and chemotherapeutic agent. *Molecular Nutrition & Food Research* 2008; 52 (Suppl 1):S103-S127.

37. Saleem M, et al. Lupeol, a fruit and vegetable based triterpene, induces apoptotic death of human pancreatic adenocarcinoma cells via inhibition of Ras signaling pathway. *Carcinogenesis* 2005; 26:1956-1964.

38. Murtaza I, et al. Suppression of cFLIP by lupeol, a dietary triter-pene, is sufficient to overcome resistance to TRAIL-mediated apoptosis in chemoresistant human pancreatic cancer cells. *Cancer Research* 2009; 69:1156–1165.

39. Saleem M, et al. Lupeol inhibits growth of highly aggressive human metastatic melanoma cells *in vitro* and *in vivo* by inducing apoptosis. *Clinical Cancer Research* 2008; 14:2119-2127.

40. Saleem M, et al. Lupeol inhibits proliferation of human prostate cancer cells by targeting beta-catenin signaling. *Carcinogenesis* 2009; 30:808-817.

41. Woyengo TA, et al. Anticancer effects of phytosterols. *European Journal of Clinical Nutrition* 2009; 63:813-820.

42. Bradford PG, Awad AB. Phytosterols as anticancer compounds. *Molecular Nutrition & Food Research* 2007; 51:161-170.

43. Wendell M, Heller AR. Anticancer actions of omega-3 fatty acids—current state and future perspectives. *Anticancer Agents in Medicinal Chemistry* 2009; 9:457-470.

44. Berquin IM, et al. Multi-targeted therapy of cancer by omega-3 fatty acids. *Cancer Letters* 2008; 269:363-377.

45. The effect of vitamin E and beta-carotene on the incidence of lung cancer and other cancers in male smokers. The Alpha-Tocopherol, Beta-Carotene Cancer Prevention Study Group. *New England Journal of Medicine* 1994; 330:1029-1035.

46. Lippman SM, et al. Effect of selenium and vitamin E on risk of prostate cancer and other cancer; the Selenium and Vitamin E Cancer Prevention Trial (SELECT). *Journal of the American Medical Association* 2009; 301:39-51.

47. Miller ER, et al. Meta-analysis: high-dosage vitamin E supple-mentation may increase all-cause mortality. *Annals of Internal Medicine* 2005; 142:37-46.

48. Albanes D, et al. Alpha-Tocopherol and beta-carotene supplements and lung cancer incidence in the alpha-tocopherol, beta-carotene cancer prevention study: effects of baseline characteristics and study compliance. *Journal of the National Cancer Institute* 1996; 88:1560-1570.

49. Virtamo J, et al. Incidence of cancer and mortality following alpha-tocopherol and beta-carotene supplementation: a postintervention follow-up. *Journal of the American Medical Association* 2003; 290:476-485.

50. Bjelakovic G, et al. Antioxidant supplements for prevention of mortality in healthy participants and patients with various diseases. *Cochrane Database of Systematic Reviews* 2008; 16:CD007176.

51. Bjelakovic G, et al. Antioxidant supplements for prevention of gastrointestinal cancers: a systematic review and meta-analysis. *Lancet* 2004; 364:1219-1228.

52. Karppi J, et al. Serum lycopene and the risk of cancer: the Kuopio Ischaemic Heart Disease Risk Factor (KIHD) study. *Annals of Epidemiology* 2009; 19:512-518.

53. Ebbing M, et al. Cancer incidence and mortality after treatment with folic acid and vitamin B12. *Journal of the American Medical Association* 2009; 302:2119-2126.

54. Ingraham BA, et al. Molecular basis of the potential of vitamin D to prevent cancer. *Current Medical Research & Opinion* 2008; 24:139-149.

55. Wei, MY, et al. Vitamin D and prevention of colorectal adenoma: a meta-analysis. *Cancer Epidemiology, Biomarkers & Prevention* 2008; 17:2958-2969.

56. Mizoue T, et al. Calcium, dairy foods, vitamin D, and colorectal cancer risk: the Fukuoka Colorectal Cancer Study. *Cancer Epidemiology, Biomarkers & Prevention* 2008; 17:2800-2807.

57. Otani T, et al. Plasma vitamin D and risk of colorectal cancer: the Japan Public Health Center-Based Prospective Study. *British Journal of Cancer* 2007; 97:446-451.

58. Wactawski-Wende J, et al. Calcium plus vitamin D supplementation and the risk of colorectal cancer. *New England Journal of Medicine* 2006; 354:684-696.

59. Grant WB, et al. An estimate of cancer mortality rate reductions in Europe and the US with 1,000 IU of oral vitamin D per day. *Recent Results in Cancer Research* 2007; 174:225-234.

60. Crew KD, et al. Association between plasma 25-hydroxyvitamin D and breast cancer risk. *Cancer Prevention Research* 2009; 2:598-604.

61. Chen P, et al. Meta-analysis of vitamin D, calcium and the prevention of breast cancer. *Breast Cancer Research & Treatment* 2009; Oct 23. [Epub ahead of print].

62. Rejnmark L, et al. Reduced prediagnostic 25-hydroxyvitamin D levels in women with breast cancer: a nested case-control study. *Cancer Epidemiology, Biomarkers & Prevention* 2009; 18:2655-2660.

63. Woo TC, et al. Pilot study: potential role of vitamin D (cholecalciferol) in patients with PSA relapse after definitive therapy. *Nutrition & Cancer* 2005; 51:32-36.

CHAPTER 11

EXERCISE & CANCER PREVENTION

Regular exercise appears to play a potentially important role in a cancer prevention lifestyle, independent of whether a person is obese or not. Based upon available clinical research data, the risk of both prostate cancer and breast cancer appear to be reduced by increased levels of physical activity, in particular.

As is the case with all public health research studies looking at disease prevention, one can always find studies that identify no apparent link between exercise and cancer prevention. However, there are multiple well-performed prospective clinical research studies that *do* strongly suggest a role for exercise in the reduction of prostate cancer and breast cancer risk. For example, a recent prospective clinical study evaluated 190 veterans who were scheduled to undergo needle biopsy of their prostate glands. Prior to undergoing their biopsies, the men were asked to complete a questionnaire related to their exercise habits. After adjusting for differences in age, race, body weight (BMI), prostate-specific antigen (PSA) level, digital rectal examination findings, family history, prior prostate biopsy history, and other prostate cancer risk factors, the researchers then assessed the incidence of prostate cancer in the biopsy specimens. They found that the men who reported even rather moderate levels of regular exercise (9 or more mets per week) had a *65 percent lower* risk of prostate cancer when compared to the men who reported the least amount of regular physical activity. Among the men who were diagnosed with prostate cancer by needle biopsy, moderate levels of regular exercise also appeared to be associated with lower grade (i.e., less aggressive) tumors [1].

A large prospective public health study, performed in Sweden, enrolled nearly 46,000 men between the ages of 45 and 79 years, and followed these men for an average of almost 10 years. Extensive personal and occupational histories were taken for all of these men. Compared with men who sat down throughout most of their workday, men who spent at least half of their workday walking or standing experienced a *20 percent lower risk* of developing prostate cancer. Moreover, each reported 30-minute per day period of daily walking or bicycling was associated with a *7 percent decrease* in the risk of developing prostate cancer (within a range of 30 to 120 minutes of walking or bicycling per day) [2].

Breast cancer risk, like prostate cancer risk, also appears to be favorably affected by regular exercise, particularly over long periods of time. A large prospective public health study, published in the prestigious *New England Journal of Medicine*, enrolled more than 25,000 women between the ages of 20 and 54 years. All of these women completed extensive health surveys, as well as questionnaires regarding their leisure-time and work activities. This very large group of women was followed for an average of nearly 14 years, during which time 351 new cases of breast cancer were diagnosed. Among the women who exercised regularly, the risk of breast cancer was *37 percent lower* when compared to the women who did not exercise. The risk of breast cancer was *decreased even further, by 72 percent*, in thin women who exercised at least 4 hours per week. As has been previously observed for men with respect to prostate cancer risk, increased levels of physical activity at work were also associated with a decreased risk of breast cancer in this large group of women [3].

Another very large prospective study, the landmark Nurses' Health Study II, which included nearly 65,000 women, also evaluated leisure-time activity levels and the risk of breast cancer in premenopausal women. After an average of 6 years of follow-up, 550 premenopausal women in this study were diagnosed with breast cancer. As with other studies, this study determined that long periods of increased physical activity were associated with a decreased risk of breast cancer. Specifically, there was a *23 percent reduction* in the risk of breast cancer among the premenopausal women who regularly engaged in the equivalent of 3.25 hours of running per week, or 13 hours of walking per week. Moreover, the earlier women began regularly exercising in their lives, the greater the cumulative protective effect of exercise in preventing breast cancer [4].

Although the association between exercise and cancer prevention appears to be strongest for prostate cancer and breast cancer, there is some evidence that other types of cancer may also be less common among people who regularly exercise. For example, an enormously large prospective public health study, the European Prospective Investigation into Cancer and Nutrition (the EPIC Study), followed more than 420,000 patient volunteers for an average of 9 years. All participants in this gigantic epidemiological study were assessed with respect to their levels of exercise and other physical activities. Diet, lifestyle, and other health-related behaviors were also surveyed. This study revealed that patients who frequently engaged in regular exercise throughout the week were *31 percent less likely* to develop stomach (gastric) cancer when compared to sedentary patients who did not exercise [5].

In another prospective public health study, from Finland, 2,560 adult male volunteers were followed for almost 17 years. Once again, increasing levels of regular physical activity were associated with decreasing levels in the risk of premature death due to cancer in these men. After adjusting for differences among these men in age, alcohol consumption, smoking, weight (BMI), and dietary habits, this study determined that moderate levels of regular exercise (at least 30 minutes per day) were associated with a *37 percent decrease* in the risk of dying of cancer (and, especially, death due to gastrointestinal tract cancers and lung cancer) [6].

References

1. Antonelli JA, et al. Exercise and prostate cancer risk in a cohort of veterans undergoing prostate needle biopsy. *Journal of Urology* 2009; 182:2226-2231. Orsini N, et al.

2. A prospective study of lifetime physical activity and prostate cancer incidence and mortality. *British Journal of Cancer* 2009; 101; 1932-1938.

3. Thune I, et al. Physical activity and the risk of breast cancer. *New England Journal of Medicine* 1997; 336:1269-1275.

4. Maruti SS, et al. A prospective study of age-specific physical activity and premenopausal breast cancer. *Journal of the National Cancer Institute* 2008; 100:728-737.

5. Huerta JM, et al. Prospective study of physical activity and risk of primary adenocarcinomas of the oesophagus and stomach in the RPIC (European Prospective Investigation into cancer and

nutrition) cohort. *Cancer Causes and Control* 2010 [Epub ahead of print].

6. Laukkanen JA, et al. Intensity of leisure-time physical activity and cancer mortality in men. *Journal of Sports Medicine* 2009 [Epub ahead of print].

CHAPTER 12

PRESCRIPTION MEDICATIONS & CANCER PREVENTION

Several classes of prescription medications have been variably associated with a decreased risk of cancer.

Selective Estrogen Receptor Modulators

A class of medications referred to as selective estrogen receptor modulators (SERMs), which includes tamoxifen and raloxifene, has been shown to reduce the risk of breast cancer in high-risk women by nearly 50 percent. SERMs will, therefore, be more extensively discussed in the expanded chapter on breast cancer.

Non-Steroidal Anti-Inflammatory Drugs

Non-steroidal anti-inflammatory drugs (NSAIDs) include aspirin, ibuprofen, naproxen, and other commonly used prescription and non-prescription pain medications. These medications have been shown to have significant cancer prevention properties, particularly against colorectal cancer. However, increasing concern regarding adverse cardiovascular effects associated with most NSAIDs (but not aspirin) has limited enthusiasm for their use as cancer prevention agents, except in patients with inherited predispositions to develop colorectal cancer [1].

Statins

The statin drugs function by blocking an enzyme known as HMG-CoA reductase, which is necessary for the creation of cholesterol in the body. Most statin drugs also have significant anti-inflammatory effects. However, the available clinical research data is mixed with respect to whether or not statin drugs significantly reduce the risk of cancer.

In a moderately large epidemiological study that included 1,953 patients with recently diagnosed colorectal cancer, and a control group of 2,015 patients without colorectal cancer, a *47 percent reduction* in the risk of colorectal cancer was observed following long-term statin use [2].

Unfortunately, the cumulative data on statin drugs as potential cancer prevention agents remains contradictory, overall. For example, in another cancer prevention study, national health care databases in Finland were utilized to evaluate nearly 1 million patients, half of whom routinely took statin drugs and half of whom did not. Following an average duration of follow-up of almost 9 years, this huge population-based public health study *did not detect any difference* in the incidence of cancer between these two groups of patients [3]. On the other hand, a large decade-long prospective French study of nearly 8,000 men revealed a *59 percent reduction* in the risk of death due to cancer in men who took statin medications (as compared to men with elevated cholesterol levels who were not taking statins) [4].

Because of the contradictory data available regarding statin medications and cancer risk, it is not currently recommended that patients be started on statin drugs solely for cancer prevention purposes.

Diabetes, Metformin & Cancer Prevention

Diabetes has been linked to an increased risk of several types of cancer. Metformin, also known as Glucophage, is widely considered as the initial treatment of choice for patients with diabetes, and especially for obese diabetics. Metformin functions primarily by reducing the production of glucose (sugar) by the liver. Several recent high-quality clinical studies of metformin have raised the intriguing possibility that this commonly prescribed medication may also reduce the risk of cancer, and cancer-associated death, in diabetic patients, in addition to lowering elevated blood sugar levels.

In one such study, 1,353 diabetic patients were prospectively followed. At the end of almost 10 years of follow-up, diabetic patients were found to have a *47 percent higher* risk of cancer-associated death than the general population. However, diabetic patients who took metformin for their diabetes experienced a whopping *57 percent reduction* in the risk of death due to cancer when compared to diabetic patients who were not taking metformin [5].

Pancreatic cancer is a particularly deadly form of cancer, and diabetes is a known risk factor for this form of cancer. A study from the M.D. Anderson Cancer Center evaluated the incidence of pancreatic cancer in diabetic patients who were receiving various treatments for diabetes, including insulin injections, insulin-releasing oral medications, and metformin. A total of 973 patients who were diagnosed with pancreatic cancer (including 259 diabetic patients) and 863 patients without pancreatic cancer (including 109 diabetic patients) were enrolled in this clinical study. Diabetic patients taking metformin were found to have a *62 percent lower risk* of developing pancreatic cancer when compared to patients who were not taking metformin. Moreover, patients who were taking insulin injections or insulin-releasing pills to treat their diabetes actually experienced an *increased* risk of developing pancreatic cancer [6].

These and other clinical studies strongly suggest that metformin significantly lowers the risk of cancer and cancer-associated death in diabetic patients (there is also data suggesting that the response of breast cancer to chemotherapy may be improved in diabetic patients who are taking metformin).

Although diabetic patients are at a higher risk of developing cancer, clinical studies suggest that metformin can reduce cancer risk in diabetics to a level that is less than what is observed in the general population. This suggests that metformin may potentially have a role as a cancer prevention medication in the general population, although its use in non-diabetic patients has not yet been extensively studied. Based upon the available clinical data, so far, some cancer experts are calling for a randomized, prospective, double-blind clinical study of metformin as a potential cancer prevention agent.

References

1. Bertagnolli MM, et al. Five-year efficacy and safety analysis of the Adenoma Prevention with Celecoxib Trial. *Cancer Prevention Research* 2009; 2:310-321.

2. Poynter, JN., et al. Statins and the risk of colorectal cancer. *New England Journal of Medicine* 2005; 352:2184–2192.

3. Haukka J, et al. Incidence of cancer and statin usage—record linkage study. *International Journal of Cancer* 2010; 126:279-284.

4.   Gardette V, et al. Ten-year all-cause mortality in presumably healthy subjects on lipid-lowering drugs (from the Prospective Epidemiological Study of Myocardial Infarction [PRIME] prospective cohort). *American Journal of Cardiology* 2009; 103:381-386.

5.   Landman GW, et al. Metformin associated with lower cancer mortality in type 2 diabetes (Zodiac-16). *Diabetes Care* 2009 [Epub ahead of print].

6.   Li D, et al. Antidiabetic therapies affect risk of pancreatic cancer. *Gastroenterology* 2009; 137:482-488.

PART II

EXPANDED CLINICAL CANCER SECTION

CHAPTER 13

INTRODUCTION

In this section, I have included a particularly detailed discussion of the top three cancer killers in the United States (and throughout much of the world). Together, lung cancer, breast cancer, and prostate cancer account for 41 percent, or nearly half, of all cancer cases, and 40 percent of all cancer deaths in the United States. These three cancers cause the combined deaths of nearly 250,000 Americans every year, and many more hundreds of thousands of people around the world each year. (Ironically, lung cancer, the most prolific cancer killer of all, is also the most preventable of all of the major cancer killers.)

CHAPTER 14

LUNG CANCER

Overview of Lung Cancer

More than 219,000 new cases of lung cancer were diagnosed in the United States in 2009, representing approximately 15 percent of all cancer diagnoses, and making lung cancer the most commonly diagnosed type of cancer in America [1]. Lung cancer also remains, by far, the most common cause of cancer-related death in the U.S., causing more than 159,000 deaths in 2009, or approximately *one-third* of all cancer-related deaths [2]. The lethality of this horrible disease is underscored by the fact that the number of deaths due to lung cancer every year is equal to 73 percent of the number of new cases diagnosed each year. (Presently, only about 10 to 15 percent of patients with lung cancer will survive 5 years beyond their initial diagnosis.)

The overall incidence of lung cancer in the United States has been gradually decreasing over the past few decades, as the proportion of the population that smokes has slowly continued to decline following the publication of the landmark Surgeon General's report on smoking in 1964. In that report, lung cancer was directly linked with smoking. However, tragically, 45 years later, lung cancer still remains the undisputed #1 cancer killer in the United States, and throughout much of the world, as well.

While the overall incidence of lung cancer and the number of annual lung cancer deaths have been slowly declining in the United States for the past decade, these favorable epidemiologic trends have been confined exclusively to the male half of the population. Over the past 4 decades, an increasing number of American women have taken up smoking and, not surprisingly, the incidence of lung cancer and the number of lung cancer deaths among women have been rising, year-after-year, as well. (Within the past 3 years, however, it appears that lung cancer deaths among women in the United States may have finally reached a plateau, although the number of newly diagnosed cases of lung cancer among U.S. women is still slowly rising.)

Much of the "credit" for sparking the decades-long epidemic of smoking and lung cancer among women can be attributed to advertising campaigns targeted specifically towards women by tobacco companies. Indeed, perhaps no other advertising campaign targeting women is better known, or more infamous, than Phillip Morris' wildly successful campaign for its Virginia Slims brand of cigarettes. This cigarette, which was intentionally manufactured with a narrower diameter and a longer length than competing brands, was introduced in 1968 with its catchy advertising hook, "You've Come a Long Way, Baby!" Unfortunately, for millions of women who became smokers in response to these socially irresponsible advertising campaigns, their long journey has ended, sadly, with diagnoses such as chronic bronchitis, emphysema, heart disease, stroke, peripheral vascular disease, and lung cancer; and in their often painful deaths from these terrible but preventable smoking-associated diseases.

Niche-advertising targeted towards young women, as exemplified by the multi-decade advertising campaign for Virginia Slims, along with changing societal attitudes in the 1960s and 1970s towards smoking among women, gave women around the world a new form of equality that they would have been far better off never having achieved. Advertisements linking smoking with female emancipation hardly conveyed the most profoundly emancipating effect of cigarettes, which was that hundreds of thousands of women could now join their smoking male counterparts in dying miserable and often prolonged deaths from a cancer that can be prevented in more than 90 percent of cases, simply by avoiding exposure to tobacco. While the incidence of smoking and lung cancer death rates among women have recently begun to plateau, more than 100,000 women were diagnosed with lung cancer in 2009, and more than 71,000 additional women died during the same year from this almost completely preventable form of cancer [3]. They also became members of a huge, but unenviable, fraternity encompassing the 500,000 men and women who die prematurely, each and every year, from completely preventable tobacco-associated diseases in the United States (and the millions more who suffer terribly, until their premature deaths, from these same preventable diseases).

Among all of the known cancer killers in the United States, none are as prolific in causing death as lung cancer, and at the same time, ironically, no other cancer is as preventable. This simple and irrefutable fact belies a public health tragedy of truly staggering dimensions. Indeed, whenever I am confronted with the casual disregard of the risks associated with smoking that many of my smoking patients express when I counsel them to quit, it never fails to upset me. Unfortunately, many smokers are predisposed to rationalizing their addiction to nicotine, and often greet my expressions of concern with responses like, "Hey, Doc, you gotta die of something!" I sometimes feel a strong urge to ask such patients to join me on my rounds through our cancer center to see the physically wasted men and women who, gasping to catch their final breaths, are dying a lingering, miserable, and yet almost completely preventable death from lung cancer, as their loved ones and physicians look on, helpless to rescue them from their terrible and irreversible fates.

More than 40 years after the direct scientific linkage between smoking and lung cancer was publicly affirmed, the enormous public health tragedy of lung cancer continues relatively unabated. As it has been for numerous decades now, lung cancer remains the undisputed heavyweight champion of cancer-associated death in the United States (the richest, most prosperous and, arguably, the most highly educated society in the history of humankind).

But there is hope that this cancer scourge can someday be defeated. In the United States, at least, the number of smokers continues to decline, having recently reached a historically low level of just under 20 percent of the total adult population at the time of this book's publication. However, as cancer quickly approaches the unfortunate distinction as the #1 cause of death throughout the world, lung cancer will continue to lead the march of new cancer deaths across our planet. In fact, the continuing rise in the number of smokers throughout much of the developing world is considered by public health experts to be the single most important factor in propelling cancer to become the greatest cause of preventable death, worldwide, in 2010. As the large tobacco conglomerates have increasingly turned their deep pockets and market-tested advertising machines away from the United States, and towards developing countries and other developed countries, the global lung cancer pandemic continues to grow each year. At the present time, an estimated 1.2 million people, or the equivalent of the entire population of Dallas, Texas, die each year around the world from smoking-associated cancers, and this number is expected to continue to rise for the foreseeable future.

Risk Factors for Lung Cancer

Tobacco & Lung Cancer Risk

It has been estimated that more than 15 *billion cigarettes are smoked around the world each day*, and that *more than 1 million deaths occur each year*, globally, due to smoking-associated cancers (many millions more die each year of smoking-associated non-cancer illnesses, as well). In the United States, alone, cigarette smoking causes a whopping *34 percent of all cancer deaths* [4].

Tobacco smoke contains an amazing variety of substances that have been proven to be carcinogenic to humans, as well as many additional chemical compounds that are highly suspected of being carcinogenic. Based upon published laboratory research, there are currently at least 62 known carcinogenic substances present in tobacco smoke, and at least 15 of these chemical substances have been directly shown to cause cancer in humans [5].

At the risk of being repetitive, lung cancer is the #1 cause of cancer death in the United States, and yet it is also the easiest cancer to prevent. In our daunting quest to rid mankind of all types of cancer, the eradication of lung cancer is an absolutely achievable goal, as more than 90 percent of all lung cancers are directly caused by smoking [6].

The lifetime risk of developing lung cancer, like other tobacco-associated diseases, is directly proportional to several well understood factors, primarily including the age at which smoking is initiated, the number of cigarettes smoked each day, and the number of years spent smoking. For example, becoming a smoker at age 15 is associated with a *doubling* of one's lifetime risk of developing lung cancer when compared to taking up smoking during adulthood [7]. Unfortunately, more than 80 percent of all smokers begin smoking during childhood or adolescence [8]. (The children of smoking parents are *5 to 7 times more likely* to, themselves, become smokers when compared to kids who have non-smoking parents.) According to recent American Lung Association statistics, more than 1,300 children and teens become new smokers each and every day in the United States, alone, and approximately *half of them will eventually die prematurely* as a direct result of smoking-associated diseases.

Smoking over a prolonged period of time, irrespective of a smoker's age at the onset of smoking, significantly increases the risk of lung cancer. Indeed, smoking one pack of cigarettes per day for 40 years is associated with nearly *twice* the lifetime risk of dying from lung cancer as is seen in smokers who have "only" smoked one pack per day for 30 years [9].

Clearly, inhaling the poly-carcinogenic combustion products of tobacco is a highly efficient way for tobacco to cause both lung cancer and chronic non-cancer lung diseases. However, despite the common perception that the use of snuff, and other forms of smokeless tobacco, is safer than smoking tobacco, the potent human carcinogens N-nitrosamines are also present, and in high concentrations, in smokeless tobacco. N-nitrosamines have been definitively linked to cancers of the lung, nasal and oral cavities, esophagus, liver, pancreas, bladder, and cervix [10].

Not only does tobacco account for more than 90 percent of all lung cancer cases, but exposure to various forms of tobacco (including exposure to second-hand smoke) has also been definitively linked to cancers of the oral and nasal cavities, larynx (voice box), esophagus, stomach, colon, rectum, liver, pancreas, ovary, cervix, prostate, bladder, and bone marrow (leukemia), among others.

Irrespective of its form, or the route of its ingestion, there simply is no safe or healthful use for tobacco [11].

Radon Gas, Ionizing Radiation & Lung Cancer Risk

Chronic exposure to radon gas is the second most common risk factor for lung cancer, and as with virtually all non-tobacco lung cancer risk factors, smokers who are chronically exposed to radon gas have an even greater risk of developing lung cancer than similarly exposed non-smokers.

Radon is a colorless, odorless, and tasteless radioactive gas that results from the natural isotopic decay of uranium. (Uranium is present, in varying concentrations, within the bedrock beneath the soil.) Radon gas easily seeps through tiny cracks in basement foundations and walls, and closed spaces within buildings can trap radon gas until it reaches concentrations that are high enough to induce lung cancer, particularly at or below ground level. Published scientific estimates regarding the percentage of lung cancer cases caused by radon gas exposure vary, but it is generally agreed that *5 to 10 percent* of all lung cancer cases are caused by radon gas.

Patients who have received radiation therapy as treatment for other cancers are also at increased risk of developing secondary cancers, including lung cancer.

Most notably, breast cancer and lymphoma patients who have previously received therapeutic radiation therapy to the chest are at increased risk of developing lung cancer, with radiation-induced lung cancers arising, on average, 5 to 10 years following completion of radiation therapy.

Even radiation exposure from routine diagnostic x-ray tests is known to cause mutations in our DNA, and can potentially cause lung cancer and other types of cancer. The increasing use of computed tomography (CT) scanners, which can subject the body to significant doses of ionizing radiation during a single examination, has also raised concerns about the potential of these scans to cause lung cancer and other types of cancer as well.

Other Environmental Risk Factors for Lung Cancer

In addition to radon gas and other sources of ionizing radiation, significant environmental exposures to asbestos, nickel, cobalt, cadmium, chromium, and diesel exhaust have also been implicated in the development of lung cancer. Moreover, smoking appears to have a synergistic cancer-causing effect when combined with exposure to asbestos, radon gas, or uranium ore. Although the precise contribution of each of these potential environmental carcinogens to the overall incidence of lung cancer is not completely understood, they are believed to account for a very small percentage of all lung cancer cases diagnosed in the United States. Smoking and radon gas, on the other hand, account for *95 to 99 percent* of all lung cancer cases in the United States, and throughout much of the world as well.

Screening for Lung Cancer

Radiographic Studies & Lung Cancer Screening: Chest X-ray & CT Scans

The ideal approach to screening for lung cancer continues to be hotly debated, as there is no scientific consensus that any of the currently available screening methods are associated with a meaningful reduction in the death rate due to this cancer. At the present time, the most commonly used screening methods are plain chest x-rays, CT scans of the chest, and sputum cytology. Among these screening exams, routine annual chest x-ray remains the most commonly ordered lung cancer screening test. The primary advantages of plain chest x-ray are its ability to detect lung tumors that are at least 1 inch (2 to 3 centimeters) in diameter and its relatively low cost.

High-resolution CT scans of the chest received an enormous boost as a lung cancer screening tool in 2006, when a group from Cornell University published their seemingly compelling clinical research data in the *New England Journal of Medicine* [12]. The authors of this research study claimed that the routine use of CT scans to screen smokers and ex-smokers resulted in remarkably improved survival rates among those patients in whom lung cancer was first detected by such scans. However, the conclusions of this study, which was the first to show any significant lung cancer survival benefit associated with early detection using CT scans, have since been called into question by the authors' revelations, in 2008 (and under pressure, I might add), that $3.6 million, or *virtually all of the funding* used to conduct this study, had been donated to the researchers by the parent company of Liggett Tobacco, a cigarette manufacturer. Further investigation into this obvious conflict of interest also revealed that the primary author of the study, Dr. Claudia Henschke, holds patents issued for the CT scanner technology utilized in this study, and from which Cornell University also apparently receives patent royalty fees. General Electric, a dominant manufacturer of CT scanners, is also listed as holding two of these same patents, and it has also recently been revealed that additional funding for this study was provided by General Electric, as well [13].

This questionable Cornell study aside, there is currently no compelling high-level clinical research data that has confirmed a significant improvement in survival among patients in whom lung cancer has been detected by radiographic screening, including the use of either plain chest x-rays or CT scans. In fact, recently, a large study of more than 3,000 asymptomatic current and former smokers, with an average follow-up of 4 years, found that, while more lung cancers were detected in the group of patients that underwent screening CT scans, and more patients in this group underwent surgery for lung cancer, there were *no subsequent survival differences* between the two groups of patient volunteers [14]. The results of this study are in keeping with the results of multiple other clinical research studies that have, so far, failed to identify any significant lung cancer survival advantage following the routine use of chest x-rays or CT scans to screen smokers and ex-smokers. At the same time, CT scans often identify nodules in the lung that, in the long run, turn out to be benign. The detection of these (benign) nodules by CT scans often leads to multiple serial CT scans over time, in an effort to monitor these small, indeterminate lung nodules, and to multiple unnecessary invasive biopsy procedures (with their attendant risks). Additionally, CT scans of the chest expose patients to significant doses of ionizing radiation, and repeated CT scans, performed in an effort to monitor indeterminate lung nodules detected by an initial CT scan, expose patients to even higher cumulative doses of radiation.

(Ionizing radiation exposure to the torso is, itself, a known risk factor for several types of cancer, including, ironically, lung cancer.)

Fortunately, a large ongoing prospective clinical research trial, the National Lung Screening Trial (NLST), may settle the controversy surrounding the impact, if any, of CT scan screening on lung cancer survival. In this study, a comparison will be made between plain chest x-rays and low-dose CT scans. The impact, if any, that each of these screening tests might have on lung cancer survival rates will be analyzed at the conclusion of this study. However, it will be several more years before the data from this clinical trial will be available for analysis. Therefore, at the present time, the American Cancer Society *does not recommend any routine radiographic tests* for the purpose of screening for lung cancer (including plain chest x-rays or CT scans), unless patients are participating in a clinical research trial such as the NLST study.

Sputum Testing for Lung Cancer

The role of sputum testing in lung cancer screening, if any, is, likewise, unclear at this time. Conventional sputum testing, or sputum cytology, involves looking at coughed-up secretions from the lungs under a microscope, in an effort to detect sloughed lung cancer cells. Unfortunately, sputum cytology is not very sensitive in detecting early lung cancers, and therefore does *not* appear to be associated with any significant clinical benefit [15]. However, newer genetically-based sputum screening tests are currently being evaluated, and some of these "molecular" tests may eventually turn out to be clinically useful. These molecular screening tests are becoming increasingly more sensitive in detecting miniscule amounts of genetic material from cancer cells that are shed into the sputum within the lungs. At the present time, however, the use of these molecular sputum tests is limited to research studies, only. (Additional clinical research will be necessary before we will know if these very expensive tests have a potential role in screening for lung cancer.)

Lung Cancer Prevention Strategies

Lifestyle & Behavioral Strategies for Lung Cancer Prevention

Among all of the cancers that are discussed in this book, none can be more easily and more effectively prevented than lung cancer, the single greatest cause of cancer-associated death in the United States (and throughout much of the world, as well). Based upon the estimates of many of the world's most prominent epidemiologists and cancer experts, at least 90 percent of lung cancer deaths in the United States can be completely prevented simply by eliminating the use of tobacco (in any form) [16]. There is no debate whatsoever when it comes to the direct link between tobacco use and lung cancer causation. Change tobacco-associated behaviors, and you will dramatically change the incidence of the #1 cancer killer throughout most of the world.

More than 80 percent of smokers start their deadly habit before or during adolescence. However, even if every adolescent on the planet could be persuaded to avoid taking up the use of tobacco, that still leaves an estimated *1.2 billion active smokers in the world* today [17]. In view of this unfortunate reality, what hope can be offered to current smokers that, if they quit, they might still significantly reduce their lifetime risk of developing lung cancer? Fortunately, there is abundant research data to call upon in this area. In one of the largest studies of its kind, a huge cohort of more than 280,000 U.S. military veterans was followed for an average duration of 26 years. This powerful clinical study revealed that the lung cancer risk of ex-smokers, when compared to those who never smoked, was *16-fold* greater during the first 5 years after quitting, and declined to a magnitude of *8-fold* greater risk 5 to 10 years after quitting. In this very large epidemiological study, the relative risk of developing lung cancer then gradually declined further, to about *2 times the risk of never-smokers*, between 10 and 30 years after giving up tobacco [18]. Thus, abstaining from smoking can indeed dramatically reduce one's risk of developing lung cancer (as well as other serious smoking-associated diseases), and the longer an ex-smoker remains tobacco-free, the lower their lung cancer risk becomes. (However, for long-term smokers, the lifetime risk of developing lung cancer after quitting never becomes as low as it is for never-smokers.)

Chronic exposure to radon gas is the (distant) #2 cause of lung cancer, and accounts for an estimated *5 to 10 percent* of all lung cancer cases. Radon gas is generated from the natural decay of uranium, a radioactive metal that is present throughout the earth's crust. Although radon gas is rather ubiquitously present throughout the environment, it tends to build up in areas at or below ground level, and especially in low-lying areas where there is poor ventilation. Uranium mines, not surprisingly, are associated with the highest levels of radon gas. (Uranium miners who also smoke are at an especially high risk of developing lung cancer due to the combined carcinogenic effects of radon gas and tobacco smoke on the tissues that line the lungs.) However, for most people, chronic exposure to radon gas occurs at home. While there is considerable geographic variation in ground-level radon gas concentrations, basements and other lower levels of homes that have been built on or near soil containing high levels of uranium can accumulate clinically significant concentrations of this colorless, odorless, and tasteless gas. In homes that are tightly sealed against the environment, as is common in areas where there are extremes of temperature throughout the year, dangerously high levels of radon gas can accumulate. Radon gas can also diffuse into groundwater, and people who rely upon wells for drinking water may, therefore, also ingest toxic levels of radon gas by drinking from radon-contaminated water sources.

The combined effects of smoking and radon gas exposure synergistically increase the likelihood of developing lung cancer, above and beyond the sum of the individual risks of each factor. In fact, the majority of lung cancer deaths associated with known radon gas exposure actually occur among smokers [19].

The only way to accurately assess radon levels in your home is through testing by a licensed radon gas testing company. As radon concentrations within a home can vary from day-to-day, most experts recommend longer term testing (i.e., optimally, more than 90 days of continuous testing), rather than the 24 to 48 hours of testing that is more commonly performed. In the United States, the Environmental Protection Agency recommends that radon gas abatement interventions be performed if the average radon gas level within a home reaches or exceeds 4 picocuries per liter (pCi/L). Radon gas abatement interventions generally involve the installation of ventilation systems in affected basements (and, sometimes, on ground-level floors as well) to prevent toxic accumulations of this carcinogenic gas. These systems range in cost from about $1,000 to $3,000 for most homes.

Additional useful information about radon gas testing and radon gas abatement can be found at http://www.epa.gov/iaq/radon and http://www.nsc.org/issues/radon/.

Diet, Nutrition, Supplements, Medications & Lung Cancer Risk

The role of diet and dietary supplements in lung cancer prevention is unclear at this time, although recent research has been very disappointing in this area. At the present time, against the backdrop of the overwhelming association of lung cancer with a completely preventable behavior (i.e., smoking), there does not appear to be any other prevention strategy on the horizon that would provide a significant improvement in lung cancer risk beyond avoiding exposure to tobacco (and excessive levels of radon gas).

There are several large, prospective, randomized lung cancer prevention research studies that have identified an *increase* in lung cancer rates (and overall mortality) following the use of certain vitamin supplements in smokers.

Therefore, the use of vitamin supplements as a strategy to reduce lung cancer risk has fallen out of favor

To date, there have been three landmark clinical research studies that have evaluated the Vitamin A derivative beta-carotene (either alone or in combination with other vitamins) as a potential lung cancer prevention agent. Each of these three research studies was a prospective, randomized, placebo-controlled clinical trial with long follow-up of large numbers of patient volunteers. These studies were developed because earlier survey-based public health studies suggested that people who consume large amounts of fruits and vegetables rich in beta-carotene appeared to have a lower risk of developing lung cancer. Other clinical studies have examined the level of beta-carotene in the blood of patient volunteers, and some of these studies have, likewise, suggested that beta-carotene might be associated with a protective effect against lung cancer. However, the data from these three landmark beta-carotene prospective clinical trials has been anything but encouraging.

The huge CARET (Beta-Carotene and Retinol Efficacy Trial) study randomized more than 18,000 volunteers to receive either pills containing beta-carotene and Vitamin A, or identical appearing placebo (sugar) pills. The study volunteers were all considered to be at high risk of developing lung cancer due to a history of smoking or/and asbestos exposure. This study was actually prematurely halted when it became evident that the group taking the beta-carotene and Vitamin A pills had already reached a *28 percent higher* incidence of lung cancer, and a *17 percent increase* in the risk of death, when compared to the group of otherwise matched volunteers who had been secretly assigned to take placebo pills. Among these volunteer patients, *current* smokers experienced the greatest risk of lung cancer and death within the group randomized to receive beta-carotene and Vitamin A supplements [20].

The second landmark lung cancer prevention trial is the ATBC (Alpha-Tocopherol Beta-Carotene Cancer Prevention Trial) study. In this large placebo-controlled randomized clinical trial, carefully matched groups of middle-aged male smokers were randomized to receive beta-carotene, Vitamin E, both vitamins, or placebo pills. Altogether, this study included more than 29,000 patient volunteers, and the duration of follow-up of these volunteers ranged from 5 to 8 years. In the ATBC trial, just as was observed in the CARET study, the men who were secretly assigned to take beta-carotene experienced an *increased* incidence of lung cancer compared to the men in the placebo group. In the beta-carotene group, the risk of lung cancer was *18 percent higher* than was observed in the group of men who did not receive beta-carotene. Likewise, the men who received beta-carotene were also *8 percent more likely to die* when compared to the men who did not receive this vitamin supplement [21].

While these two high-level randomized prospective clinical trials both revealed that beta-carotene supplementation appears to be harmful in active or recent smokers, beta-carotene's effects on cancer prevention have also been recently studied in non-smokers as well. The enormous Physicians' Health Study, composed of male physician volunteers (the great majority of whom were non-smokers), evaluated beta-carotene as a potential cancer prevention agent. Over 22,000 male physicians were followed for an average of 13 years in this prospective clinical trial. The Physicians' Health Study revealed absolutely *no* increase *or* decrease in the risk of lung cancer, prostate cancer, or colon cancer associated with beta-carotene supplementation in this study's predominantly nonsmoking volunteers [22]. Therefore, the data from this very large prospective study of mostly non-smoking men failed to show any impact of beta-carotene supplements on the risk of the three most commonly occurring cancers in men.

Thus, while much less rigorous public health studies had previously suggested that beta-carotene might reduce the risk of lung cancer, three huge prospective, double-blinded, randomized clinical trials have failed to show *any* benefit from beta-carotene supplementation in reducing the risk of lung cancer, either in smokers or non-smokers. Moreover, the risk of lung cancer actually appears to be *increased* (as well as the overall risk of death) among active or recent smokers who take beta-carotene supplements.

Finally, in 2003, an exhaustive review was performed of previously published clinical lung cancer research studies looking at beta-carotene and Vitamin E, encompassing a total of nearly 110,000 research volunteers. *This comprehensive review concluded that there was no convincing scientific evidence that either of these supplements offered any protection against lung cancer in otherwise healthy people* [23].

While there are a few small and low-powered studies that have identified specific dietary supplements and vitamins as potential lung cancer prevention agents, none of these research studies have the scientific and statistical power to compete with the large randomized controlled trials that I have already summarized. Moreover, the results of many of these smaller and less rigorous studies contradict each other, as well. Broccoli and other cruciferous vegetables, grapes, red wine, green tea, soy protein, cholesterol-lowering statin drugs, various Vitamin A derivatives, Vitamin C, and grapefruit juice, among other dietary agents, have all been suggested to have potential lung cancer prevention properties based upon small, low-powered studies, particularly among non-smokers [24-34].

Unfortunately, there are currently no vitamins or other dietary supplements that can be formally recommended for the prevention of lung cancer, at least based upon data from multiple large, high-level, prospective, randomized clinical trials. Perhaps future prospective, randomized clinical trials will identify one or more dietary supplements that can actually reduce the risk of lung cancer in humans, but there is no compelling available data in this regard at the present time. So, for now anyway, the best strategy available to reduce one's risk of lung cancer, as well as many other cancers, is to eat a well-balanced diet that is rich in fresh fruits and vegetables (and low in red meats and saturated fats), and to completely abstain from exposure to tobacco, in any form [35].

In summary, I end this section on lung cancer much as I began my discussion of this awful disease. Among all of the cancer killers that affect humans, at least 95 percent of all cases of lung cancer, which remains the #1 cause of cancer death in the United States, can be **prevented** simply by avoiding exposure to tobacco and radon gas. *Thus, in my view, the greatest irony within the entire field of cancer prevention is that the most prolific cancer killer of our time is also the most preventable of all of the major types of cancer.*

References

1.   Cancer Facts & Figures 2009, The American Cancer Society.

2.   Cancer Facts & Figures 2009, The American Cancer Society.

3.   Cancer Facts & Figures 2009, The American Cancer Society.

4.   Mackay J, Eriksen M. The tobacco atlas. Geneva: World Health Organization, 2002:24.

5.   International Agency for Research on Cancer. Tobacco smoke and involuntary smoking. IARC Monographs on the Evaluation of Carcinogenic Risks to Humans, vol. 83. Lyon, France: IARC, 2004:53.

6.   International Agency for Research on Cancer. Tobacco smoke and involuntary smoking. IARC Monographs on the Evaluation of Carcinogenic Risks to Humans, vol. 83. Lyon, France: IARC, 2004:1179.

7.   Peto R, Darby S, Deo H, et al. Smoking, smoking cessation, and lung cancer in the UK since 1950: combination of national statistics with two case-control studies. *British Medical Journal* 2000; 321:323-329.

8.   Rainio SU, et al. Evolution of the association between parental and child smoking in Finland between 1977 and 2005. *Preventive Medicine* 2008; 46:565-571.

9.   Alberg AJ, Samet JM. Epidemiology of lung cancer. *Chest* 2003; 123(1 Suppl):21S.

10.   International Agency for Research on Cancer. Smokeless tobacco and tobacco-specific nitrosamines. IARC Monographs on the Evaluation of Carcinogenic Risks to Humans, vol. 89. Lyon, France: IARC, 2007.

11.   Stewart SL, et al. Surveillance for cancers associated with tobacco use—United States, 1999-2004. Morbidity and Mortality Weekly Report (MMWR) Surveillance Summary 2008; 57:1-33.

12.   Henschke CI, et al. Survival of Patients with Stage I Lung Cancer Detected on CT Screening. *New England Journal of Medicine* 2006; 355:1763-1771.

13.   *Cancer Letter* (2008; 34[2].

14.   Bach PB, et al. Computed tomography screening and lung cancer outcomes. *Journal of the American Medical Association* 2007; 297:953-961.

15.   Bach PB, et al. Screening for lung cancer: a review of the current literature. *Chest.* 2003; 123(1 Suppl):72S-82S.

16.   Cigarette Smoking Among Adults — United States, 2007. Morbidity and Mortality Weekly Report (MMWR) 2008; 57:1221-1226.

17. Mackay J, Eriksen M. The Tobacco Atlas. Geneva: World Health Organization, 2002:24.

18. Hrubec Z, McLaughlin JK. Former cigarette smoking and mortality among US veterans: a 26-year follow-up, 1954–1980. In: Burns DM, Garfinkel L, Samet J, editors. Changes in cigarette-related disease risks and their implication for prevention and control. Bethesda, MD: US Government Printing office; 1997, p. 5010.

19. Darby S, et al. Radon in homes and risk of lung cancer: collaborative analysis of individual data from 13 European case-control studies. *British Medical Journal* 2005; 330:223-238.

20. Omenn GS, et al. Risk factors for lung cancer and for intervention effects in CARET, the Beta-Carotene and Retinol Efficacy Trial. *Journal of the National Cancer Institute* 1996; 88:1550-1559.

21. The effect of vitamin E and beta carotene on the incidence of lung cancer and other cancers in male smokers. *New England Journal of Medicine* 1994; 220:1029-1035.

22. Cook NR et al., Effects of beta-carotene supplementation on cancer incidence by baseline characteristics in the Physicians' Health Study (United States). *Cancer Causes and Control* 200; 11:617-626.

23. Caraballoso M, et al. Drugs for preventing lung cancer in healthy people. *Cochrane Database of Systematic Reviews* 2003; CD002141.

24. Brennan P, et al. Effect of cruciferous vegetables on lung cancer in patients stratified by genetic status; a mendellian randomization approach. *Lancet* 2005; 366:1558-1560.

25. Farwell WR, et al. The association between statins and cancer incidence in a veterans population. *Journal of the National Cancer Institute* 2008; 100:124-139.

26. Aziz MH, et al. Cancer chemoprevention by resveratrol: in vitro and in vivo studies and the underlying mechanisms (review). *International Journal of Oncology* 2003; 23:17-28.

27. Kuoppala J, et al. Statins and cancer: A systematic review and meta-analysis. *European Journal of Cancer* 2008; 44:2122-2132.

28. Mahabir S, et al. Dietary alpha-, beta-, gamma-, and delta-tocopherols in lung cancer risk. *International Journal of Cancer* 2008; 123:1173-1180.

29. Le Marchand L. et al. Intake of flavonoids and lung cancer. *Journal of the National Cancer Institute* 2000; 92:154-160.

30. Arts IC. A review of the epidemiological evidence on tea, flavonoids, and lung cancer. *Journal of Nutrition* 2008; 138:1561S-1566S.

31. Li Q, et al. Green tea consumption and lung cancer risk: the Ohsaki study. *British Journal of Cancer* 2008; 99:1179-1184.

32. Gray J, et al. Lung cancer chemoprevention: ACCP evidence-based clinical practice guidelines (2nd edition). *Chest* 2007; 132:56S-68S.

33. Mayne ST, et al. Dietary beta-carotene and lung cancer risk in U.S. nonsmokers. *Journal of the National Cancer Institute* 1994; 86:33-38.

34. Cohen V & Khuri FR. Chemoprevention of lung cancer. *Current Opinions in Pulmonary Medicine* 2004; 10:279-283.

35. Gonzalez CA. The European Prospective Investigation into Cancer and Nutrition (EPIC). *Public Health Nutrition* 2006; 9:124-126.

CHAPTER 15

BREAST CANCER

Overview of Breast Cancer

Excluding minor skin cancers, breast cancer is the single most common type of cancer among women, and the second most common cancer-related cause of death in women (lung cancer still kills nearly twice as many women in the United States every year as does breast cancer). Based upon American Cancer Society data, there were more than 192,000 new cases of breast cancer diagnosed in 2009, accounting for 27 percent of all cancer cases among women. In 2009, nearly 41,000 women died from this common form of cancer [1]. Moreover, 62,000 additional women were also diagnosed with precancerous changes of the breast in 2009, including ductal carcinoma *in situ* (DCIS), and the less common lobular carcinoma *in situ* (LCIS).

It is important to note that men can also develop—and die from—breast cancer too. An estimated 2,000 men in the United States were diagnosed with breast cancer in 2009, and nearly 500 men died of this disease in 2009 [2].

Beginning in 2003, the incidence of breast cancer, and the number of breast cancer deaths, finally began to decline after decades of gradual and sustained annual increases. The reasons for the previous *rise* in breast cancer incidence have been the subject of intense debate within the scientific and medical communities for many years. Similarly, the more recently observed *declines* in new breast cancer cases, and in the death rate due to breast cancer, have also stimulated considerable recent debate, as well. (I'll have more to say about this debate, momentarily.)

In terms of cancer prevention and treatment research, no other type of cancer has benefited so enormously from the social activism of its victims as has breast cancer. Bernadine Healy, the first woman to head the prestigious National Institutes of Health (1991 to 1993) has estimated that between 1991 and 2005, American taxpayers funded over $10 billion in breast cancer research, or more than 8 times as many research dollars as were invested in researching the considerably more lethal cancers of the lung, pancreas, ovary, and liver, combined [3].

Over the past 40 years, numerous grassroots and organized women's health advocacy groups have compelled both public and private research funding agencies to provide an enormous pool of research dollars for the study of breast cancer prevention, detection, and treatment. In cancer centers across the country every year, hundreds of millions of dollars in research funds are being invested in improving early detection strategies for breast cancer, and in finding more effective treatments. This enormous sum of research dollars flows from regional and national government-funded public health agencies, and from private breast cancer advocacy foundations like the Susan G. Komen For the Cure Foundation, the Avon Foundation, and many others. (Indeed, before the Federal Government began to offer large-scale funding for breast cancer research, critical research funding was often available *only* through private breast cancer advocacy groups and foundations in the United States.) Unfortunately, with large National Cancer Institute research funding cuts looming in our current deficit-ridden economy, the demand for increased breast cancer research funding by private philanthropic groups is already apparent.

In my view, advocacy groups for other types of cancer have a great deal to learn from the countless millions of women (and men) who have successfully advocated for adequate funding for breast, ovarian, and uterine cancer research. Although the disproportionately high number of research dollars invested in breast cancer research (compared to research funding for other types of cancer) has occasionally given rise to complaints by some cancer research advocates, out of the tremendous volume of scientific and clinical data that has resulted from breast cancer research over the past 40 years, we have also been able to significantly improve our understanding of the intricate biology of many other types of cancer, as well.

Breast Cancer Risk Factors

The list of known risk factors associated with breast cancer is, by far, the largest among all types of cancer. Therefore, there are also multiple opportunities available to reduce the risk of this disease.

Gender, Age & Breast Cancer Risk

The two most important risk factors for breast cancer are female gender and increasing age (approximately two-thirds of all breast cancer cases occur in women over the age of 50). While these two risk factors cannot, obviously, be modified, many other breast cancer risk factors *can* be significantly modified, as I shall discuss.

Family History & Hereditary Breast Cancer Syndromes

As with many other types of cancer, family history and inheritance play a significant role in a person's risk of developing breast cancer (although it should be remembered that 70 percent of women newly diagnosed with breast cancer have no known history of the disease in their families). If you have a history of breast cancer in your family, your lifetime risk of breast cancer may be increased, as well. Indeed, having a mother, sister, or daughter with breast cancer nearly *doubles* a woman's lifetime risk of breast cancer, and having two or more immediate family members with breast cancer increases a woman's lifetime risk to *nearly 5 times that of the general population.*

At the present time, fewer than 10 percent of all breast cancer cases are associated with mutations of genes known to cause hereditary breast cancer syndromes. Among the half dozen or so genes linked to hereditary breast cancer syndromes so far, the BRCA1 and BRCA2 genes are the most common. Certain mutations of either of these genes are associated with a 70 to 80 percent lifetime risk of developing breast cancer, as well as a 30 to 50 percent lifetime risk of ovarian and peritoneal cancers. (BRCA1 and BRCA2 gene mutations are also associated with an increased risk of breast cancer and prostate cancer in men who carry these "deleterious" mutations.)

It is important to remember that *both* women *and* men can carry BRCA1 and BRCA2 cancer gene mutations, and can therefore pass them on to *both* their daughters *and* sons. Because almost all inherited cancer gene mutations, including the BRCA1 and BRCA2 gene mutations, are passed on to successive generations through an autosomal dominant type of inheritance pattern, there is a roughly 50 percent chance that each son and daughter of an affected parent will inherit the same cancer gene mutation. Thus, it is important to remember that BRCA1 and BRCA2 gene mutations can be passed down to females from their male parents. As only about 5 percent of all men who are affected with BRCA1 or BRCA2 gene mutations will actually go on to develop breast cancer (although up to 25 percent of affected men will develop prostate cancer), women who inherit BRCA1 or BRCA2 gene mutations from their fathers may unknowingly be at high risk of developing breast and ovarian cancer, as there may be no previous history of breast or ovarian cancer in such families. In fact, a surprising number of physicians are also unaware of the clinical implications of autosomal dominant cancer gene inheritance, and many doctors fail to ask female patients about a family history of BRCA-associated cancers other than female breast cancer.

The percentage of women in the general population who carry BRCA1 and BRCA2 gene mutations is not entirely clear. Most clinical studies looking at the percentage, or prevalence, of women carrying these gene mutations have focused almost exclusively on patients who have already been diagnosed with early-onset breast cancers. Even among women with early-onset breast cancers, however, the prevalence of these hereditary breast and ovarian cancer syndrome gene mutations varies considerably among different ethnic and geographical populations of women. Fortunately, though, there are two particularly useful BRCA gene mutation research studies that have recently been published.

In a large clinical study of Caucasian and African-American women between the ages of 35 and 65, nearly 1,700 women with breast cancer and 674 women without breast cancer underwent genetic testing for both BRCA1 and BRCA2 gene mutations [4]. Overall, approximately 2 percent of the women with early-onset breast cancer carried a BRCA1 gene mutation and 2 percent carried a BRCA2 gene mutation. BRCA1 gene mutations were more common in Caucasian breast cancer patients (2.9 percent) than African-American patients (1.4 percent); and slightly more than 10 percent of the Jewish breast cancer patients carried a BRCA1 gene mutation, versus 2 percent of the non-Jewish patients. In contrast, the prevalence of BRCA2 mutations did not significantly differ between Caucasian and African-American women with breast cancer, nor between Jewish and non-Jewish breast cancer patients.

Among the breast cancer patients without any family history of breast cancer, 1.9 percent carried a BRCA1 gene mutation. However, the prevalence of BRCA1 mutations among the women with breast cancer increased to 3.1 percent with an associated history of breast cancer among one or more second degree relatives (e.g., aunts, uncles, half-siblings, grandparents, and grandchildren), and increased, further, to 5.6 percent, with any history of breast cancer among first degree relatives (e.g., parents, siblings, and children). Jewish ancestry, the diagnosis of breast cancer before age 45 in one or more relatives, bilateral breast cancer in one or more relatives, 3 or more relatives with breast cancer, or ovarian cancer in one or more relatives (especially when combined with a family history of breast cancer) were all risk factors that particularly increased the likelihood of BRCA1 gene mutations in this group of 1,700 breast cancer patients. In contrast to BRCA1 mutations, the two risk factors that best predicted the presence of BRCA2 gene mutations were an early age at breast cancer diagnosis and, similarly, having relatives who were also diagnosed with breast cancer at an early age. Among the 674 women volunteers who did *not* have breast cancer, 0.04 percent were found to have BRCA1 gene mutations, and 0.4 percent were discovered to have BRCA2 gene mutations.

In a second multiethnic study, more than 1,200 early-onset female breast cancer patients participating in a familial breast cancer registry in California were assessed for the presence of BRCA1 gene mutations. All of these women, who were diagnosed with breast cancer before the age of 65, underwent testing for BRCA1 gene mutations. Among Ashkenazi Jewish patients, 8 percent had BRCA1 gene mutations, while only 2 percent of the remaining non-Hispanic Caucasian women were found to carry BRCA1 mutations. Among Hispanic patients, nearly 4 percent carried BRCA1 gene mutations; and among African-American women with breast cancer diagnosed before the age of 65, only about 1 percent carried BRCA1 mutations. Finally, among Asian women with early-onset breast cancer, only 0.5 percent carried BRCA1 gene mutations [5].

As these two large clinical studies have clearly shown, BRCA1 and BRCA2 gene mutations are significantly more likely to be present when there is a family history of breast cancer and/or ovarian cancer. However, families have recently tended to become much more fragmented in our modern society, and many of us have only limited knowledge of the health histories of our extended families. The clinical importance of this fact of modern life was emphasized in a recent study of more than 300 women who were diagnosed with breast cancer before the age of 50. In this study, half of the women were unable to provide a complete family history, while the other half were able to give a complete family history. Among the early-onset breast cancer patients who were able to provide a complete family history, *5 percent* tested positive for either BRCA1 or BRCA2 gene mutations. However, *14 percent* of the young women who were unable to provide a complete family health history tested positive for BRCA1 or BRCA2 cancer gene mutations. Thus, in this group of women with early-onset breast cancer, BRCA1 and BRCA2 gene mutations were almost *3 times more common* among women with early-onset breast cancer who were not able provide a detailed family health history [6]. As we used to say when I was a medical student, "History is King," and when one is trying to ascertain potential genetic contributions to an individual patient's cancer risk profile, a thorough and complete family history can be critically important.

In addition to the BRCA1 and BRCA2 genes, other gene mutations associated with an increased risk of breast cancer have been described, although these gene mutations are exceedingly rare in the general population. Li-Fraumeni Syndrome, which is most commonly caused by mutations in the P53 gene, is associated with a 60 percent lifetime risk of developing breast cancer, as well as an increased risk of brain tumors, leukemia, sarcomas of the soft tissues and bone, adrenal gland tumors, melanoma, and other benign and malignant tumors. Another very rare inherited syndrome associated with breast cancer is the Peutz-Jeghers Syndrome, which is caused by mutations in the STK11/LKB1 gene. This syndrome is associated with intestinal polyps, and a lifetime breast cancer risk of 50 to 55 percent. This prolific hereditary cancer syndrome is also associated with an increased risk of cancers of the lung, stomach, small intestine, colon, rectum, pancreas, cervix, ovary, uterus, and testicles. Cowden's Syndrome, another very rare inherited syndrome, is most commonly caused by mutations in the PTEN gene (an even rarer variant of PTEN gene mutation, and also linked to an increased risk of breast cancer, is the Bannayan–Riley–Ruvalcaba syndrome). Women affected with Cowden's Syndrome have a 25 to 50 percent lifetime risk of developing breast cancer, as well as a very high risk of benign tumors of the skin, bones, brain, eyes, and urinary tract. Cowden's Syndrome is also associated with an increased risk of thyroid cancer, as well. Very rare mutations of two other genes, ATM and CHEK2, have also been associated with an increased lifetime risk of breast cancer.

As with most hereditary cancer syndromes, gene mutations associated with an increased risk of breast cancer not only increase a woman's overall lifetime risk of breast cancer, but are also associated with the onset of breast cancer at an earlier than usual age, as well.

Hormones & Breast Cancer Risk

The female sex hormones estrogen and progesterone are thought to play a critical role in the development of the great majority of breast cancers, and this helps to explain why breast cancer is nearly 100 times more common in women than in men, and why a woman's cumulative lifetime exposure to female sex hormones affects her lifetime breast cancer risk. For example, the early onset of menstrual periods (menarche) and the late onset of menopause are known risk factors for breast cancer, as is the use of hormone replacement therapy (HRT) pills for relief of menopausal symptoms (and, especially, the combination estrogen and progesterone HRT pills that are prescribed for women who still have their uterus). The long-term use of oral contraceptive pills may also slightly increase a woman's lifetime risk of breast cancer, although the risk of ovarian cancer appears to be reduced at the same time. Fortunately, this very small increase in the risk of breast cancer appears to subside after discontinuing oral contraceptives.

Delaying full-term pregnancy until after age 30, or not having children at all, also appears to *increase* a woman's risk of developing breast cancer. For those women who do bear children, *not* breastfeeding has also been shown to *increase* the risk of breast cancer. Childbirth during young adulthood, and breastfeeding, both appear to modify the cells that line the milk ducts and milk glands of the female breast, rendering them less likely to transform into breast cancer cells later in life. Hormonal factors appear to be involved in all of these reproduction-related breast cancer risk factors, although the precise mechanisms are not entirely understood at this time.

Hormone replacement therapy (HRT) medications, taken for the symptoms of menopause, have been available since the 1940s. HRT medications became enormously popular in the United States, and throughout the developed world, in the 1960s, as a result of both the women's emancipation movement and the publication of a peculiar little paperback book by a Manhattan gynecologist. In this book, *Feminine Forever*, gynecologist Dr. Robert A. Wilson capitalized on the blossoming women's equality and sexual liberation movements, and upon the growing global emphasis on women's health issues that resulted from these movements, by writing a book that would dramatically change the perceptions of menopause in the United States, and, indeed, throughout much of the developed world. As the number of prescriptions for HRT rose following the 1966 publication of *Feminine Forever* (and its characterization of menopause as a pathological state of lost femininity and mental deterioration), the number of new cases of breast cancer also rose in lock-step. Despite the near-universal knowledge that the cumulative, lifelong extent of exposure to the primary female sex hormones (estrogen and progesterone) is associated with the lifetime risk of developing breast cancer, the dominant Big Pharma company in the HRT market aggressively discounted any proposed links between HRT medications and the rising incidence of breast cancer. (The extent to which the dangerous health effects of HRT medications were suppressed by this drug company, including this company's covert collusion with Dr. Wilson in the publication of *Feminine Forever*, is the subject of my next book, "Hormone Replacement Therapy (HRT) & the Breast Cancer Epidemic.")

In July of 2002, the Journal of the American Medical Association (JAMA) published a landmark public health study that powerfully indicted HRT as a specific and significant risk factor for breast cancer. This prospective, randomized, placebo-controlled study evaluated 16,608 postmenopausal women who were taking either hormone replacement pills or placebo pills (sugar pills). A total of 8,506 women took tablets containing estrogen and progestin, the two female "sex hormones," while 8,102 women took identical-appearing placebo pills. (Progestin is added to HRT in women who still have their uterus, as "unopposed" estrogen HRT is known to *increase* the risk of uterine cancer.)

The Women's Health Initiative study was originally designed to last 8.5 years, but was halted after only 5 years when the trial's data and safety monitoring board determined that the health risks associated with HRT were excessively high. Following a complete analysis of the data, this study found that the use of estrogen and progestin HRT *increased the relative risk of breast cancer by 26%*, and that this increased risk begins to develop within 4 years of starting HRT [7].

At this time, I counsel *all* postmenopausal women to avoid hormone replacement therapy. For patients who are already taking HRT, I strongly urge them to gradually wean themselves off of these drugs with the assistance of their physicians.

Prior Breast Cancer, Dense Breasts & Other Breast Abnormalities

A prior diagnosis of breast cancer, by itself, significantly increases a woman's lifelong risk of subsequently developing a *new* breast cancer (in *either* breast). Indeed, a previous history of breast cancer is associated with *3 to 4 times the risk* of developing another breast cancer when compared to the general population (currently, the average American woman has an 8 to 9 percent lifetime risk of developing breast cancer).

Increased breast density has also recently been discovered to be a risk factor for breast cancer. Women with especially dense breast tissue may not only harbor small cancers that can be difficult to detect by standard breast cancer screening tests, but their very dense and glandular breasts are also more likely to develop breast cancers, as well.

Women with certain types of benign breast lesions are also at an increased risk of developing breast cancer. Completely benign lesions of the breast that are known to increase a woman's risk of breast cancer include ductal or lobular hyperplasia (an overgrowth of otherwise normal breast cells), as well as other so-called "benign proliferative" lesions of the breast. These other benign breast lesions include ductal papillomas, benign fibrous tumors called fibroadenomas, sclerosing adenosis, and radial scars. These benign lesions have been estimated to increase the lifetime risk of breast cancer from 1.5 to 3 times that of the general population, even when no atypical "precancerous" changes in the cells of these lesions are identified under the microscope.

When cells begin to appear abnormal, or atypical, under the pathologist's microscope, then there is a greater likelihood that the process of transformation from a completely normal breast cell, to something more closely resembling a cancer cell, has already begun. An overgrowth of atypical milk duct or milk gland cells (atypical ductal hyperplasia, or ADH, and atypical lobular hyperplasia, or ALH, respectively) is associated with *3 to 5 times* the lifetime risk of developing breast cancer when compared to the general population, while ADH or ALH *plus* an extensive family history of breast cancer may increase a woman's lifetime risk of breast cancer by as much as *9 to 10 times* that of the general population's risk (and also greatly increases the likelihood that a BRCA1 or BRCA2 gene mutation is present).

Ductal carcinoma *in situ* (DCIS) and lobular carcinoma *in situ* (LCIS) are breast lesions that represent true precancerous changes of the cells that line the milk ducts and milk glands (respectively), and the presence of these lesions, alone, can increase a woman's lifetime risk of developing invasive breast cancer to as high as *15 to 30 percent.*

Race, Ethnicity & Breast Cancer Risk

Race and ethnicity, at least in the United States, appear to have a rather modest effect on breast cancer risk, except among recent immigrants from countries that have a very low risk of breast cancer. For example, multiple studies have shown that recent immigrants from Japan (where the incidence of breast cancer has, historically, been much lower than in the United States) continue to experience low rates of breast cancer, while each successive generation of their American-born daughters and granddaughters experiences an incidence of breast cancer that more closely approximates that of the US population as a whole. (This repeated observation is strong evidence that environmental and lifestyle factors are likely at work in increasing the incidence of breast cancer here in the United States.)

Within the United States, however, breast cancer is somewhat more common in Caucasians when compared to Asian, Hispanic and Native-American women. At the same time, while African-American women are slightly *less* likely to develop breast cancer when compared to Caucasian women, they are *more likely to die* from their breast cancers, probably due to a combination of biologically more aggressive forms of cancer in some African-American patients, and delays in diagnosis in others.

Prior Radiation Treatment & Breast Cancer Risk

Prior radiation therapy to the chest area, particularly during childhood and adolescence, is also associated with an increased lifetime risk of breast cancer. Older methods of radiation treatment for Hodgkin's lymphoma often sub-jected teens and young adults to extensive irradiation of the breasts. Several long-term studies of these patients have shown a spike in the incidence of breast cancer 10 to 20 years after completion of radiation treatment for Hodgkin's lymphoma.

Obesity & Breast Cancer Risk

Obesity has long been linked to an increased risk of postmenopausal breast can-cer, most likely due to the increased production of estrogen and other hor-mones by excess fatty tissue. Moreover, obesity that is centered around the abdominal area (central, or truncal, obesity) appears to be associated with a greater risk of breast cancer than the more common female pattern of hip, but-tock, and thigh obesity. *Although estimates vary, most experts believe that obesity increases a woman's relative risk of developing breast cancer by 20 to 50 percent, with most of this increased risk arising during the postmenopausal years* [8, 9].

Alcohol & Breast Cancer Risk

An under-appreciated risk factor for breast cancer is alcohol consumption. Numerous studies have definitively linked regular alcohol consumption with a significantly *increased* risk of breast cancer in women. (Even moderate alcohol intake increases production of the female sex hormones that are asso-ciated with the most common type of breast cancer.) Drinking more than 2 alcoholic drinks per day, in particular, appears to increase a woman's life-time risk of breast cancer by *1.5 to 2 times (50 to 100 percent)* above that of the general population (1 alcoholic drink is considered to be a mixed drink, a glass of wine, or a glass of beer) [10-12].

Even one alcoholic drink per day has been shown, by a large prospective clin-ical trial, to be associated with a small but significant increase in the lifetime risk of breast cancer [13]. A recent meta-analysis based on data from 53 dif-ferent clinical research studies concluded that alcohol consumption increased the relative risk of developing breast cancer by *7 percent for each daily single serving of alcohol consumed.* Furthermore, the results from this large meta-analysis suggest that about *4 percent* of all breast cancers in developed countries may be caused directly by alcohol consumption. Finally, this landmark study also found that *even a single alcoholic beverage per day* was associated with a sta-tistically significant increase in the risk of developing breast cancer [14].

Increased alcohol intake has also been linked to cancers of the pancreas, liver, ovary, oral cavity, larynx, esophagus, colon, and rectum.

Diet & Other Environmental Breast Cancer Risk Factors

Dietary factors other than alcohol appear to play an important role in breast cancer risk, as well. While the data on saturated fat intake has been both weak and contradictory with respect to breast cancer risk, there are several high quality prospective clinical studies suggesting that red meat consumption, specifically, increases one's risk of developing breast cancer (red meat and processed meats have also been linked to an increased risk of cancers of the esophagus, stomach, colon, rectum, prostate, pancreas, ovary, and other organs) [15, 16]. Given the overwhelming clinical data also linking red meat consumption with an increased risk of cardiovascular disease and other serious illnesses, dramatically reducing the intake of red meat and processed meats is an important health strategy on several different levels, including cancer risk reduction.

There are other potential dietary and environmental risk factors for breast cancer that are not fully understood yet. Unfortunately, there is no high level clinical research available at this time with which to fully validate these potential additional risk factors. However, for the sake of completeness in my discussion of breast cancer risk factors, some of these *possible* additional breast cancer risk factors include exposure to chemicals in the environment that have estrogen-like properties (e.g., DDT), plant-derived foods that have estrogen-like properties, and chronic sleep deprivation. I cannot stress strongly enough, however, that until high quality clinical research data becomes available regarding these *possible* breast cancer risk factors, their potential role in determining breast cancer risk, if any, cannot be fully ascertained at this time.

Stress & Breast Cancer Risk

The role of stress as a potential risk factor for breast cancer is unclear at this time. One large public health study has identified a mild increase in breast cancer risk among women working full-time (but not part-time) in highly stressful jobs, while another large women's health epidemiological study did not find any association between stress at work and breast cancer risk [17, 18]. However, as the immune system plays an important role in cancer surveillance and prevention, chronic stress cannot be completely ruled out as a possible risk factor for breast cancer and, perhaps, for other types of cancer as well.

Smoking & Breast Cancer Risk

There is considerable public health research data suggesting that both active and passive smoking may *significantly increase the risk* of developing breast cancer. As just one example, a very large public health study (the California Teachers Study), which followed more than 57,000 women for an average of 10 years, found that women who were regularly exposed to secondhand smoke experienced a *26 percent increase* in the risk of developing breast cancer [19].

Screening for Breast Cancer

Mammograms, Ultrasound & Breast Self-Examination

The optimal approach to breast cancer screening is the subject of ongoing debate at this time. While there have been a miniscule number of research studies (particularly from Scandinavia) that have called into question the benefit of regular screening mammograms, overwhelmingly, the data collected by high quality clinical research studies around the world continues to show that mammograms save lives by diagnosing breast cancer at an earlier, and hence more curable, stage. Despite the ongoing debate about optimal breast cancer screening strategies, there are well established, evidence-based breast cancer screening guidelines available for both the general population and high-risk patients.

For the general population, regular clinical breast examinations should be performed, starting at age 20, by at least one of a woman's primary physicians. While experts disagree on the ideal screening interval for women in their 20s and 30s, a clinical breast examination every 2 to 3 years is reasonable as long as no unusual breast cancer risk factors or breast abnormalities are present. Once a woman reaches the age of 40, however, screening recommendations for breast cancer change considerably, based upon the current consensus by breast cancer experts. For women 40 years and above, annual clinical breast examinations should be performed by physicians experienced in examining the female breast.

The controversy surrounding the ideal "age-at-onset" and frequency of screening mammograms was, once again, in the news as this book was being written and published. In November 2009, the U.S. Preventive Services Task Force (USPSTF), an agency of the U.S. Department of Health and Human Services, roiled the breast cancer community with its new recommendation that routine screening mammograms should be started at age 50 (instead of beginning at age 40, as had previously been recommended), and then every 2 years thereafter. At the time of publication of this book, in the summer of 2010, these USPSTF recommendations were still being rejected by most major breast cancer advocacy groups and breast cancer clinical experts, including the American Cancer Society, the Susan B. Komen Foundation, and the American College of Obstetricians and Gynecologists. (Tellingly, even the administration of President Barack Obama quickly distanced itself from the USPSTF recommendations, following their release.) At this time, most breast cancer experts, including those at the American Cancer Society, continue to recommend that an initial screening mammogram be performed in *all* women who are at average risk of developing breast cancer once they reach the age of 40, and then every year thereafter.

In November 2009, the American Cancer Society released a statement in response to the USPSTF's new guidelines, which read, in part:

"The USPSTF says that screening 1,339 women in their 50s to save one life makes screening worthwhile in that age group. Yet USPSTF also says screening 1,904 women ages 40 to 49 in order to save one life is not worthwhile. The American Cancer Society feels that in both cases, the lifesaving benefits of screening outweigh any potential harms. Surveys of women show that they are aware of these limitations, and also place high value on detecting breast cancer early."

There are also ongoing debates regarding the role of routine screening mammograms in elderly women (variously defined as 65 years of age or older, or 70 years of age or older). While some experts have debated the clinical value of routine mammograms in elderly women, I, like most cancer experts, continue to recommend regular annual mammograms for *all* women at or above 40 years of age, as long as they are otherwise in sufficiently good health to tolerate treatment should a breast cancer be discovered.

It is very important to remember that mammograms, like all medical tests, are not perfect. Approximately 10 to 15 percent of all breast cancers are missed by mammograms, and so patients with any suspicious changes in their breasts, even in the presence of a normal mammogram, should seek evaluation from a physician experienced in caring for breast disorders. (These clinically suspicious breast changes include a new breast lump, dimpling of the breast skin, nipple retraction, a persistent rash involving the nipple, and nipple discharge, and, especially, blood-tinged nipple discharge.)

In women younger than 35 years of age, and in all women with very dense breasts, mammograms are much less sensitive. Therefore, your doctor may suggest an ultrasound examination of the breast if he or she is concerned about any potential breast abnormalities (mammograms may or may not be ordered at the same time in women under the age of 40). Ultrasound examinations may also prove useful in women without dense breast tissue, in some cases, as well (for example, ultrasound imaging is very helpful in delineating benign cysts of the breast from more suspicious breast lesions). When performed together, ultrasound and mammographic imaging of the breast increases breast cancer screening accuracy to approximately 85 percent. (When it comes to clinical tests, unfortunately, virtually no diagnostic test offers 100 percent accuracy.)

While all current breast cancer screening tests have significant limitations, and none will detect 100 percent of all breast cancers, high-quality research has repeatedly confirmed that current breast cancer screening recommendations do, in fact, save lives. In fact an enormous and recently published British study of nearly 27,000 breast cancer patients compared 10-year survival rates between women who were diagnosed with breast cancer as a result of routine breast cancer screening imaging tests and those who were diagnosed only after a visible or palpable breast lump appeared. In this study, the women who were diagnosed with breast cancer as a result of routine annual breast screening tests were *32 percent less likely to die of breast cancer* within 10 years of diagnosis when compared to the women who were diagnosed only after their breast cancers finally became visible or palpable [20].

The topic of breast self-examination (BSE) remains more controversial than mammography, following the recent publication of several clinical studies that revealed no apparent improvement in breast cancer survival rates among women performing BSE. However, although purely anecdotal, both I and many other cancer physicians can easily recall *many* cases of breast cancer that were first detected by women (or by their partners) while performing BSE. Although the current clinical research evidence has not, in general, found a strong association between BSE and a woman's lifetime risk of dying of breast cancer, I continue to recommend BSE to most of my women patients. As there is no evidence that performing monthly BSE causes any harm, and as my own clinical experience over the past 20 years, albeit anecdotal, includes many instances where BSE findings resulted in a new diagnosis of breast cancer, I remain an advocate of BSE. However, among women with especially lumpy breasts, BSE may occasionally engender more anxiety and confusion than reassurance. If you are one of these women, then you should discuss the pros and cons of BSE further with your health care provider. If you do choose to perform BSE, it is also advisable that you have your BSE technique assessed and critiqued by a health care provider who has experience in performing clinical breast examinations.

Magnetic Resonance Imaging (MRI)

Magnetic resonance imaging (MRI) of the breast is increasingly being used to evaluate women who are at high risk of developing breast cancer, women with extremely dense breast tissue (which is, itself, a risk factor for breast cancer), women who have indeterminate findings on mammograms or breast ultrasound imaging, and women who have recently been diagnosed with breast cancer. Unlike mammograms, MRI scans do not use radiation to create images. Instead, a very powerful magnet is used to create detailed images of both breasts. The sensitivity of MRI breast imaging is significantly greater than that of mammography and breast ultrasound, with most recent clinical studies suggesting that 90 to 95 percent of breast cancers can be detected by current generation MRI machines. (The sensitivity of MRI in detecting the most common *precancerous* lesion of the breast, DCIS, actually approaches 100 percent in some studies.) But, unfortunately, there are also potential downsides associated with MRI breast imaging as well. While the sensitivity of MRI surpasses other forms of standard breast imaging at this time, the "specificity" of MRI breast imaging still remains a challenge due to MRI's high "false-positive" rate. Although improvements in MRI technology are constantly being made, at the present time, between 15 and 30 percent of breast abnormalities detected by current generation MRI machines will be proven, after biopsy, to be benign lesions. A second limitation that argues against the widespread use of MRI imaging as a routine breast cancer screening tool is the cost and efficiency of MRI scanning. MRI machines are hugely expensive, and each breast MRI examination can take an hour, and sometimes longer. Most community hospitals have a single MRI machine (some larger academic centers may have two or more MRI machines, although these additional machines are often used to perform clinical research). Because of the enormous cost and "throughput" challenges that are currently associated with MRI imaging of the breast, in addition to its relatively high false-positive rate, routine breast cancer screening using MRI imaging is not feasible at this time.

According to the American Cancer Society's recently revised breast cancer screening guidelines, MRI should be considered for screening high-risk women for breast cancer. However, in view of the limitations and expense associated with breast MRI, recent clinical research data, presented at the 2008 San Antonio Breast Cancer Symposium, has suggested that high-risk women may also significantly benefit from alternating between mammograms and breast MRI scans during their annual breast cancer screening examinations [21].

Based upon recently updated recommendations, women with the following risk factors are considered to have a *high lifetime risk* of developing breast cancer, and these women should at least consider undergoing breast imaging with MRI every year, or every other year:

- A calculated lifetime risk of breast cancer of at least 20 percent, according to validated breast cancer risk assessment tools such as the Gail model, the Claus model, the Tyrer-Cuzick model, or the BRCAPRO model.

- The confirmed presence of BRCA1 or BRCA2 gene mutations; or the presence of BRCA1 or BRCA2 gene mutations in a parent, brother, sister, or child of any woman who has not, herself, undergone BRCA1 and BRCA2 gene testing.

- The presence of a hereditary breast cancer syndrome other than BRCA1 or BRCA2 mutations; or a parent, brother, sister or child with one of these inherited syndromes. These inherited cancer syndromes include Li-Fraumeni Syndrome, Peutz-Jeghers Syndrome, Cowden's Syndrome, Bannayan-Riley-Ruvalcaba Syndrome, ataxia-telangiectasia syndrome, or mutations of the CHEK2 gene.

- A prior history of undergoing radiation therapy to the chest area between 10 and 30 years of age.

Women with the following risk factors are considered to be at a moderate lifetime risk of developing breast cancer, and may also be considered for MRI breast screening:

- A calculated lifetime risk of breast cancer of 15 percent to 20 percent, according to validated breast cancer risk assessment tools, such as the Gail model, the Claus model, the Tyrer-Cuzick model, or the BRCAPRO model.

- A personal history of breast cancer, ductal carcinoma in situ (DCIS), lobular carcinoma in situ (LCIS), atypical ductal hyperplasia (ADH), or atypical lobular hyperplasia (ALH).

- Extremely dense breasts (based upon mammogram findings).

Additionally, the American Cancer Society offers the following recommendations regarding MRI breast imaging for cancer screening purposes:

- If MRI is used, it should be in addition to, and not instead of, a screening mammogram (while MRI is more sensitive than mammography, MRI imaging can still miss some breast cancers that would otherwise be detected by a mammogram).

- For most women at high risk of developing breast cancer, annual screening with MRI and mammography should begin at age 30 years, and continue for as long as a woman is in good health. However, the clinical research evidence for this recommendation is rather limited, and so the age at which high-risk women begin breast cancer screening should be based upon discussions between patients and their health care providers, and should take into account each patient's individual health-related factors.

Finally, I would like to add the following observations regarding the use of breast cancer risk assessment tools, and the selection of an imaging facility for MRI scans of the breast:

- Several validated risk assessment tools, such as BRCAPRO, the Gail model, the Claus model, and the Tyrer-Cuzick model, can help to estimate a woman's lifetime risk of developing breast cancer. However, it is very important to remember that the results of these assessment tools are only estimates, and that each of these assessment tools may actually provide a different breast cancer risk estimate for an individual woman. (None of these risk assessment models can provide precise individual risk assessments for every single woman.) However, these risk assessment tools have been shown to accurately identify women who are at sufficiently increased risk of developing breast cancer to justify more stringent screening measures, as well as to stratify patients who should at least consider taking hormone-blocking medications (chemoprevention), or undergo prophylactic surgery, to reduce their lifetime risk of developing breast cancer.

- Women who have been advised to undergo breast MRI should choose a facility that also has the capability to perform needle biopsies using the MRI machine, as 5 to 7 percent of all breast abnormalities that are revealed by an MRI machine will be undetectable using other types of breast imaging exams.

Breast cancer is the single most common cancer that affects women, and the second most common cause of cancer-related death in women (lung cancer remains the most common cause of cancer-associated death in both men and women). While routine breast cancer screening is an anxiety-producing experience for some women, fortunately, more than 80 percent of all breast abnormalities that are identified by routine annual screening exams turn out to be benign lesions. By following the breast cancer screening guidelines that I have outlined in this chapter, women can significantly reduce their risk of dying from this common form of cancer.

Breast Cancer Prevention Strategies

Obesity, Exercise & Breast Cancer Prevention

In addition to following recommended breast cancer screening guidelines to reduce your lifetime risk of dying of breast cancer, you can take proactive steps, starting today, to reduce your risk of developing breast cancer.

Avoiding obesity is an important cancer prevention strategy for many types of cancer, including breast cancer. Not only has obesity been definitively linked to an increased risk of breast cancer, but obesity also increases the risk of cancers of the esophagus, stomach, small intestine, colon, rectum, pancreas, kidney, prostate gland, bladder, uterus, and ovaries, as well. Obesity has also been directly linked to an increased risk of heart disease and heart attacks (myocardial infarction), congestive heart failure, high blood pressure, stroke, diabetes, gallstones, arthritis, and other serious illnesses. Therefore, maintaining a healthy body weight can provide you with tremendous overall health benefits, including a reduction in your risk of developing breast cancer, as well as other types of cancer.

A landmark prospective public health study, the National Institutes of Health-AARP Diet and Health Study, followed more than 99,000 women for an average of 4 years. Women who gained 100 pounds or more after age 18 (up to age 50) were found to have *more than twice the risk* of developing breast cancer when compared to women who remained at a stable weight after age 18 [22].

There is also abundant clinical research data suggesting that 4 to 5 hours of moderate exercise per week can *reduce* a woman's lifetime risk of breast cancer *by 30 to 40 percent*, and that this protective effect of increased physical activity against breast cancer is, itself, separate and distinct from a woman's level of obesity [23-27].

For additional information on the role of exercise in breast cancer prevention, please review Chapter 11 (**Exercise & Cancer Prevention**).

Pregnancy, Breastfeeding & Breast Cancer Prevention

For women who are planning to start a family, a significant reduction in the lifetime risk of breast cancer can be achieved by having children before 30 years of age. And, as if there were not already enough good reasons to breastfeed your baby, there is solid research data showing that the longer a woman breastfeeds, cumulatively, the lower her breast cancer risk becomes. Recently, a huge review of nearly 50 previously published women's health research studies, from around the world, was performed. Altogether, these epidemiological studies evaluated more than 50,000 women with breast cancer and nearly 100,000 women without a history of breast cancer. This enormous clinical review study found that the *relative* risk of developing breast cancer *decreased by 7 percent* following each live birth, and by *more than 4 percent* for every 12 months that a woman (cumulatively) breastfed her babies. An especially compelling finding of this study was that women in both developing and developed countries experienced the same degree of breast cancer risk reduction after giving birth, and after breastfeeding their babies [28].

Although the exact mechanisms whereby full-term pregnancies and breast-feeding reduce breast cancer risk are still unclear, microscopic changes in the anatomy of the milk glands and milk ducts have been documented following childbirth, and after prolonged breastfeeding, and these changes appear to be linked with a decreased predisposition of breast cells to subsequently transform into breast cancer cells. Indeed, in view of the much higher prevalence of breastfeeding, and the simultaneously lower incidence of breast cancer, in less developed countries, prolonged breastfeeding has been proposed as one of several possible explanations for the lower incidence of breast cancer observed in less developed countries when compared to highly industrialized countries like the United States. (Decreased use of HRT medications in developing countries is another likely explanation.)

Diet & Breast Cancer Prevention

Before I review the clinical research data related to nutrition and breast cancer prevention, I must, once again, emphasize that, for much of the past 40 to 50 years, the overwhelming majority of research looking at the role of diet, nutrition, and dietary supplements in cancer risk and cancer prevention has been based upon relatively low-powered research methods. The bulk of these studies have relied upon patient surveys, the treatment of cancer cells growing in culture dishes, and the use of human tumor cells implanted into mice with defective immune systems; and all of these methodologies provide relatively low levels of clinical research evidence. However, these types of research studies are favored by researchers because they are quick and relatively cheap to perform, unlike the laborious and hugely expensive prospective, randomized, controlled clinical trials that provide "gold standard" Level 1 clinical evidence.

Unfortunately, however, what appears to work in cancer cells that are happily growing in an artificial nutrient broth, or in human tumors implanted into mice with nonfunctional immune systems, often does not work in human beings when subjected to large, high-quality, randomized, placebo-controlled, blinded, prospective human research trials. In fact, *most of the time*, the positive findings of these less rigorous preclinical studies are *not* upheld by more powerful prospective human research trials. For example, recent large and well-conducted prospective, randomized cancer prevention trials have reported their results with regards to several popular vitamins and other nutritional supplements, following decades of much lower level research studies in these areas. Unfortunately, many of these very large randomized, controlled, prospective clinical trials have failed to identify any apparent cancer prevention effect associated with specific vitamins and other commonly hyped dietary supplements. Worse yet, as I have already discussed in the chapter on lung cancer prevention, some vitamin supplements may actually be *harmful*, at least to some groups of people, if taken for prolonged periods of time, and may even *increase* the risk of the very same cancers that they were previously believed to prevent!

Although randomized, controlled human research trials remain the "gold standard" method of performing clinical research, these large multi-institutional research trials are very complex, and they are enormously expensive to perform. Thus, there is still an important role for less rigorous methods of cancer prevention research, as these relatively low-powered studies can still serve an important role in rapidly and inexpensively screening potentially promising cancer prevention strategies, which can then be further evaluated by prospective, randomized, controlled clinical trials.

As I have previously mentioned in other chapters, the frequent intake of red meat (and high-fat diets, in general) has been linked to an increased risk of cancers of the breast, esophagus, colon, rectum, pancreas, and other organs (as well as to an increased risk of cardiovascular disease) [29]. At the same time, there is also epidemiological data suggesting that cooking with monounsaturated cooking oils, and with olive oil and canola oil in particular, may also help to reduce the risk of breast cancer (although some studies have failed to confirm this finding) [30, 31]. Based upon available research evidence, however, eliminating unnecessary fat from one's diet, and making sparing use of monounsaturated cooking oils, may further decrease your risk of breast cancer (as well as other types of cancer) and cardiovascular disease.

In another prospective dietary study, from Italy, nearly 9,000 women were followed for almost 10 years, and detailed dietary surveys were performed. In this large group of women, following a Mediterranean Diet rich in fruits, vegetables, and olive oil was associated with a *35 percent decrease* in the risk of breast cancer when compared to women who consumed a typical western diet that included the frequent consumption of meat and other sources of fat, and starches (and only small amounts of fruits, vegetables, and whole grains). Given the extensive available research data associating obesity with an increased risk of breast cancer, it is not surprising that this study also noted a whopping *50 percent reduction* in the risk of breast cancer among *thin* women who regularly consumed a diet rich in raw, fresh vegetables, and olive oil, and very little meat or starches. Moreover, in this study, women who remained overweight did not significantly reduce their risk of breast cancer, even when they consumed a healthy vegetable-rich diet [32].

Clinical studies in the United States have also confirmed a link between high-fat diets and breast cancer risk. Perhaps the most important of these studies is the enormous National Institutes of Health-AARP Diet and Health Study. This huge prospective study included 188,736 postmenopausal women who were followed for an average of 4.4 years, and all of these women completed a detailed 124-item food frequency questionnaire. Women who consumed 20 percent, or less, of their daily calories in the form of fat were *11 percent less likely* to develop breast cancer when compared to women who consumed 40 percent of their daily caloric intake in the form of fat. As the follow-up duration of this huge cohort of study volunteers is still very early, it is likely that additional follow-up of these women will reveal an even higher risk of breast cancer among the women volunteers who regularly consume high-fat diets [33].

Another dietary survey-based study in the United States evaluated nearly 4,000 American women, and identified a *35 percent decrease* in the risk of breast cancer among women who consumed diets low in fat when compared to women who regularly consumed diets rich in fats (and saturated fat, in particular) [34].

While fresh fruits and vegetables are known to be beneficial in other important health-related respects, the data on the breast cancer prevention impact of fresh fruit and vegetable intake, *alone*, remains mixed. For example, several large prospective clinical trials have failed to show a significant effect of fruit and vegetable intake, *alone,* on breast cancer risk [35]. However, following a Mediterranean Diet featuring fruits and vegetables rich in *flavonoids* and *resveratrol* was found to be associated with a *significant decrease* in the risk of breast cancer in one large Italian public health study [36].

Introduction to Vitamins, Supplements & Breast Cancer Prevention

Based upon the results of recent large and highly-powered randomized, controlled, prospective human research trials, the role of most vitamins, and other dietary or "nutritional" supplements, in the prevention of breast cancer is unclear at this time.

While there are some vitamins and micronutrients that may still hold promise as potential cancer prevention agents in human, as I have discussed throughout this book, the recent data coming out of large and well-conducted prospective clinical trials has been rather disappointing, particularly with respect to that once most promising category of cancer prevention nutrients, the "antioxidant vitamins."

Vitamin D, Calcium & Breast Cancer Prevention

One of the most disappointing recent studies in the area of vitamins and breast cancer prevention is a large double-blinded, placebo-controlled, prospective clinical trial that evaluated Vitamin D and calcium supplements, as well as Vitamin D levels in the blood, in more than 2,000 postmenopausal women who participated in the enormous Women's Health Initiative Study. After an average of 7 years of follow-up, the researchers in this study did not identify any difference in the incidence of breast cancer between the group of women who were secretly randomized to receive Vitamin D and calcium supplements and the group of women who received identical placebo (sugar) pills. Moreover, unlike previous public health studies, higher levels of Vitamin D in the blood also did not appear to offer any protection against breast cancer, either [37]. The results of this study are particularly disappointing, as multiple prior epidemiological studies have strongly suggested a modest-to-moderate reduction in breast cancer incidence among women with high levels of Vitamin D and calcium in their diet, and higher levels of Vitamin D in their blood [38, 39].

However, before abandoning all hope that Vitamin D and calcium supplements have any potentially favorable effect on breast cancer risk, I should point out that there are at least three important limitations of this particular prospective study. First, some study participants took Vitamin D and calcium supplements on their own, outside of the randomization scheme of the study. Secondly, the daily Vitamin D dose of 400 International Units (IU) per day used in this study is significantly lower than the 1,000 to 2,000 IU Vitamin D daily doses that have typically been found to favorably influence cancer risk in other clinical research studies. Thirdly, the average duration of patient follow-up in this study, although relatively long at 7 years, may not yet be adequate to reveal potentially modest breast cancer prevention effects associated with long-term Vitamin D and calcium supplementation. Therefore, it may require an additional period of observation of the patient volunteers in this study before the final word is in regarding Vitamin D and calcium supplements, and their role, if any, in breast cancer prevention.

Despite the disappointing findings of the Women's Health Initiative study, there remains a significant amount of clinical research data available to at least suggest that higher levels of Vitamin D in the blood might still be associated with a reduced the risk of developing breast cancer (and other cancers, as well). For example, in one case-control study, blood levels of Vitamin D were measured in more than 1,000 breast cancer patients and more than 1,000 age-matched control patients without breast cancer. Blood levels of Vitamin D above 40 nanograms per milliliter (ng/ml) were associated with a *44 percent observed decrease* in the risk of breast cancer (and a *54 percent level of decreased* breast cancer risk in postmenopausal women, specifically) when compared with the women who had decreased levels of Vitamin D in their blood [40]. Similarly, a meta-analysis of 26 previously published Vitamin D studies found that high levels of Vitamin D in the blood were associated with a *45 percent reduction* in the incidence of breast cancer. (Higher blood levels of calcium were also associated with a *19 percent reduction* in the risk of breast cancer) [41]. Finally, yet a third case-control breast cancer study that evaluated Vitamin D levels in the blood also indentified a remarkably similar *48 percent decrease* in the risk of breast cancer associated with higher Vitamin D levels in the blood [42].

Although it is still unclear, at this time, whether or not Vitamin D supplementation can reduce a woman's lifetime risk of developing breast cancer, Vitamin D and calcium supplements, when taken in the recommended doses, are still very important for maintaining skeletal health, and also appear to reduce the risk of colorectal cancer and cardiovascular disease, as well. Prior to initiating Vitamin D and calcium supplementation, however, you should first check with your physician to be sure that you do not have any health conditions that might be worsened by these supplements. (I should also note that the World Health Organization is currently reviewing existing Vitamin D and calcium intake guidelines in view of the emerging clinical research data regarding these supplements, and I anticipate that the current recommended daily intake of these nutrients will likely be increased in the near future.)

Folic acid, Vitamin B6, and Vitamin B12 & Breast Cancer Prevention

Folic acid, Vitamin B6, and Vitamin B12 have, variably, been touted as breast cancer prevention supplements. Unfortunately, once again, newer prospective, randomized clinical trials have not confirmed the favorable findings of earlier and much less rigorous research studies involving these vitamin supplements. Recently, a large prospective clinical trial randomized more than 5,000 women to receive either placebo (sugar) pills or combined supplements of folic acid, Vitamin B6, and Vitamin B12 [43]. Following an average observation period of 7 years, there was absolutely no difference observed in the incidence of breast cancer between either group of women. While additional supplementation with folic acid, Vitamin B6, and Vitamin B12 was not associated with any reduction in breast cancer risk in this study, it is important to note that many processed foods are already routinely enriched with these same vitamins and, therefore, a modest breast cancer prevention risk associated with these supplements, if present, might have been overlooked by this study. Moreover, most breast cancers show up later in life and grow relatively slowly. Therefore, the 7-year average follow-up of these women volunteers may be insufficient to identify any early breast cancer prevention trends that might eventually arise from folic acid, Vitamin B6 or Vitamin B12 supplementation. Nonetheless, there is currently no available high-level clinical research data supporting a breast cancer prevention role for these particular vitamins.

Vitamin A, Beta-Carotene, Lycopene & Breast Cancer Prevention

Despite previous low-level research suggesting potential breast cancer inhibiting effects associated with Vitamin A, beta-carotene, lycopene and other natural or synthetic Vitamin A derivatives, there is no high-level prospective human research currently available to conclusively suggest that members of the Vitamin A family, when taken as dietary supplements, can significantly reduce one's risk of developing breast cancer.

Soy Isoflavones & Breast Cancer Prevention

Soy isoflavones, such as genistein, and other so-called phytoestrogens, have recently developed an enormous following around the world as possible breast cancer prevention aids (and as treatments for the symptoms of menopause, as well). Early interest in soy protein, and other plant-derived substances with weak estrogen-like effects, was originally stimulated by observations that women in East Asia tend to have a much lower incidence of breast cancer than women in Western countries. Among the many epidemiological and genetic factors that might explain this difference, the increased dietary intake of soy-bean-derived products, and especially tofu, in many Asian countries has been particularly noted by researchers with an interest in breast cancer prevention and treatment.

Unfortunately, although there is considerable epidemiological data supporting dietary soy-based foods as a potential breast cancer prevention agent, most of the available clinical research data in this area is derived from relatively low-level research studies, and this data has often been contradictory [44]. Some of these contradictory research findings may have resulted from the apparently contradictory biological effects that soy isoflavones appear to have when breast cancer cells are exposed to differing concentrations of these phytoestrogens. Multiple laboratory studies have shown that by varying the concentration of soy-derived isoflavones added to human breast cancer cells growing in a culture dish, breast cancer cells can be made to grow, alternately, either faster or slower. This dose-dependent "mixed agonist and antagonist" effect of soy isoflavones on estrogen receptors within the body's cells (including both benign and malignant human breast cells) complicates our understanding of the potential benefits (or risks) that might be associated with soy foods in the context of breast cancer prevention. Nonetheless, there is a reasonable body of research data, although not at a very high level, suggesting that soy foods may, indeed, slightly reduce a woman's lifetime risk of developing breast cancer, *especially when consumed before puberty or during early adolescence* [45-48].

However, until long-term randomized, placebo-controlled, prospective clinical trials have been completed in humans, my advice to female patients is to include soy-based foods and other phytoestrogens into their diets in moderation only, particularly after they pass through adolescence. In view of the ability of soy isoflavones to *increase* the growth of estrogen-sensitive breast cancer cells, at least under certain laboratory conditions, I generally advise women who are at high risk of developing breast cancer, or who have a personal history of breast cancer (or other estrogen-dependent cancers, including cancers of the ovary and uterus), to avoid these products altogether, at least until we have higher level clinical research data suggesting that these products are safe for them to consume. Fortunately, there are several ongoing prospective, randomized clinical research trials that are evaluating soy isoflavone supplements in women who are at increased risk of developing breast cancer, and in women with a prior history of breast cancer.

Green Tea (Catechins) & Breast Cancer Prevention

As with the majority of other published research looking at the effects of dietary products in disease prevention, the effects of green tea on breast cancer risk have mostly been studied using relatively weak survey-based public health studies. To date, there have been no prospective, placebo-controlled, randomized clinical trials that have comprehensively evaluated green tea as a breast cancer prevention agent, although there are multiple laboratory studies demonstrating that green tea extracts are toxic to breast cancer cells growing in a culture dish.

In looking at the available human research data, multiple epidemiological studies have, so far, revealed inconsistent findings, with most studies of Asian women revealing no apparent association between green tea consumption and breast cancer risk [49]. However, there are a few low-powered public health studies that have suggested a potential reduction in breast cancer incidence among women *who drink very large amounts* of green tea on a daily basis (in at least one Chinese study, the greatest breast cancer reduction benefit was achieved in women who consumed *at least 5 cups of green tea per day!*) [50, 51].

Virtually all of the green tea studies that have published favorable results, however, suffer from the limitations and biases inherent in case cohort studies and retrospective studies, and so definitive conclusions regarding green tea as a potential breast cancer prevention aid cannot be reached at this time.

Resveratrol & Breast Cancer Prevention

Resveratrol, which belongs to a class of antioxidant and anti-inflammatory compounds known as plant-derived polyphenols, has been the subject of a great deal of research, mostly in the area of cardiovascular medicine. Resveratrol is naturally abundant in red grapes, grape seeds, berries, peanuts, and red wine, and is thought by many experts to be one of the more important constituents of the so-called Mediterranean Diet, which has long been associated with improved cardiovascular health and a decreased risk of developing cancer. Recently, laboratory studies have identified apparent anti-cancer effects associated with resveratrol when this polyphenol is added to human breast cancer cells growing in a culture dish [52, 53].

A case-control study that evaluated 369 women with breast cancer and 602 women without breast cancer identified an apparent *61 percent reduction* in the risk of developing breast cancer among women with the highest self-reported intake of resveratrol (when compared to women with very low resveratrol intake). Interestingly, in this study, grapes appeared to be the source of resveratrol most strongly associated with a decreased breast cancer risk, while red wine intake, which is also rich in resveratrol, did not appear to reduce the risk of developing breast cancer [54]. Once again, however, I must note that the findings of relatively low-powered research methods, such as the case-control methodology used in this study, are often reversed when prospective, randomized, placebo-controlled clinical research trials are performed.

As with several other polyphenolic compounds, resveratrol does exhibit some weak estrogen-like properties, and so women with a history of estrogen dependent cancers, including cancers of the breast, ovary, and uterus, should be aware that, at least theoretically, large doses of resveratrol could potentially stimulate the growth of breast cancer and other estrogen-dependent types of cancer.

While it is not currently known if oral supplementation with resveratrol can significantly reduce the risk of cancer in humans, including breast cancer, several prospective randomized, placebo-controlled clinical cancer prevention research trials are already underway, with resveratrol, at this time.

Pomegranate Juice & Breast Cancer Prevention

Pomegranate juice is also rich in plant-derived polyphenols, and has been the subject of considerable recent cancer prevention research. However, as with the sparse data regarding resveratrol, the evidence supporting pomegranate juice as a potential breast cancer prevention aid is limited to cell culture and animal model studies in the laboratory. However, several of these low-level studies have demonstrated apparent anti-cancer effects following treatment of human and mouse breast cancer cells with pomegranate juice extracts [55]. Although there is currently no human research data available to support a breast cancer prevention role for pomegranate juice, given the favorable safety profile of pomegranate juice, it is probably safe to consume in moderate amounts (approximately 8 ounces per day). However, if you are taking cholesterol-lowering medications, or other prescription medications, you should check with your physician prior to regularly adding pomegranate juice to your diet, as pomegranate juice consumption has been occasionally linked to increased levels of statin drugs in the blood (as well as increased levels of other medications). Also, due to its high acidity, most brands of pomegranate juice contain a considerable amount of added sugar.

Sulforaphane (Cruciferous Vegetables) & Breast Cancer Prevention

In an intriguing study performed in China, 337 women were evaluated for dietary intake of cruciferous vegetables (also known as brassica vegetables), as well as soy foods and other foods that have been variably associated with breast cancer risk. An important feature of this study was the direct measurement of the metabolic byproducts of cruciferous vegetable isothiocyanates (thought to be the active anti-cancer compounds in these vegetables) in the urine of these women. After adjusting for all other known breast cancer risk factors in this group of women volunteers, high levels of isothiocyanate metabolites in the urine were correlated with a significantly reduced risk of breast cancer in a dose-dependent manner. The women with the highest levels of urinary isothiocyanates were found to be *50 percent less* likely to develop breast cancer when compared to the women with the lowest amounts of these metabolic byproducts of cruciferous vegetables in their urine. Moreover, this apparent protective effect of cruciferous vegetables against breast cancer appeared to apply equally to *both* premenopausal and postmenopausal women [56].

A recently published public health study from Singapore evaluated the impact of the regular intake of vegetables, fruit, and soy foods on the risk of breast cancer within the large Chinese population in that country. This large prospective epidemiological study, which began in 1993, included more than 34,000 women. All of the 34,018 women in this study underwent a detailed evaluation of their diets when they entered into this prospective public health study. Among this very large group of women, 629 new cases of breast cancer were diagnosed during the course of this still ongoing study.

Based upon their dietary patterns, the women participating in this large epidemiological study were divided into two groups. The first group consisted of women who regularly consumed cruciferous vegetables, fruit, and tofu. The second group of women generally favored meat and starchy foods (such as dim sum), and consumed far fewer portions of vegetables, fruit, and tofu when compared to the first group.

The results of this study indicated that *increasing levels* of vegetable, fruit and tofu intake were associated with a *significant decrease* in breast cancer risk in postmenopausal women. Among the postmenopausal women reporting the highest levels of intake of these foods, there was a *30 percent observed reduction* in the risk of breast cancer when compared to the women who rarely ate these healthy foods. Among the postmenopausal women who frequently consumed cruciferous vegetables, fruit, and tofu, and who were observed for 5 or more years in this study, the apparent reduction in the risk of breast cancer grew even stronger, as these women were found to be *43 percent less likely* to develop breast cancer when compared to women who rarely consumed cruciferous vegetables, fruit, and tofu in their diets [57].

Taken together, these two clinical studies suggest that both cruciferous vegetables and soy-derived foods (such as tofu) *may* reduce the risk of breast cancer.

Flaxseed & Breast Cancer Prevention

Because flaxseed lignans are thought to selectively both mimic and inhibit the effects of estrogen (as with soy isoflavones), there has been particular interest in these natural dietary compounds as potential breast cancer prevention agents. There is, in fact, laboratory-based evidence that flaxseed lignans are able to selectively inhibit important chemical pathways used by breast cancer cells to grow and spread. In one such study, human breast cancer tumors were implanted into laboratory mice, which were then split into two groups. The control group of mice received normal mice chow, while the experimental group of mice received a diet composed of 10 percent flaxseed. This study revealed that flaxseed lignans significantly decreased vascular endothelial growth factor (VEGF) production within the implanted human breast cancer tumors [58]. This is a potentially important finding, as VEGF is a critical cancer-associated protein that allows for tumor formation and growth by stimulating the sprouting of new blood vessels that are, in turn, necessary to support tumors as they enlarge. (As with the findings of other laboratory-based cancer prevention studies, however, it will be necessary to conduct a prospective clinical research trial to assess whether or not flaxseed supplements are also effective in preventing breast cancer in humans.)

Omega-3 Fatty Acids & Breast Cancer Prevention

In a novel laboratory study performed on breast cancer cells, fish oil appeared to increase the activity of a gene (PTEN) known to enhance cancer cell death, while also simultaneously inhibiting other genes associated with breast cancer cell growth [59]. These effects were observed after using fish oil to treat human breast cancer cells growing in cell culture dishes, and in specially-bred immune-compromised laboratory mice that had been implanted with human breast cancer tumors.

In one recent clinical study, 358 women with newly diagnosed breast cancer, and 360 women without breast cancer, underwent dietary surveys to assess their intake of fish and dietary fish oil supplements. Among the premenopausal women who regularly consumed the greatest amount of fish and fish oil in their diet, there was an observed (and whopping) *81 percent reduction* in the risk of breast cancer. Among the postmenopausal women who consumed the greatest amount of fish and omega-3 fatty acid supplements in their diet, the risk of breast cancer was *73 percent lower* than what was observed among women who consumed the least amount of fish and fish oil supplements [60].

As has been shown in thousands of prior research studies using cultured cancer cells or laboratory animals, or dietary surveys in humans, there is no guarantee that these same findings will be validated by high-quality prospective, randomized, placebo-controlled clinical research trials. Still, given the proven cardiovascular benefits associated with a diet rich in oily coldwater fish, and with omega-3 fatty acids derived from plant-based sources as well, there would appear to be little downside to incorporating moderate amounts of omega-3 fatty acids into one's diet.

Finally, as I have mentioned previously, just because a supplement is "natural" does not mean that it is non-toxic. Excessive fish intake can expose patients to elevated levels of mercury and other heavy metals. Additionally, high levels of omega-3 fatty acids can also thin the blood to the point where excessive bleeding can occur with minor injuries or surgical procedures. Finally, increased intake of omega-3 fatty acids can be toxic to some patients with underlying kidney disease. Therefore, I strongly recommend that patients check with their primary physician before initiating new dietary supplements of any kind.

Curcumin & Breast Cancer Prevention

Curcumin, a derivative of the spice turmeric (also known as curry powder), has been shown to inhibit the growth and spread of many types of cancer cells, including human breast cancer cells growing in laboratory dishes and in laboratory animals [61]. However, in other studies, curcumin has also been associated with toxic effects at higher doses, and may even *increase* the risk of tumor formation under some conditions [62]. Because of these potential adverse effects, it is unclear, at the present time, whether or not curcumin should be routinely used as a breast cancer prevention agent. However, curcumin should certainly be further studied as a potential breast cancer prevention agent through well-controlled prospective, randomized human clinical trials.

Korean Seaweed ("Gim") & Breast Cancer Prevention

A seaweed popularly consumed in South Korea (genus *Porphyra*, also known as "gim," in Korean) has recently been studied as a potential breast cancer prevention agent. A total of 362 newly diagnosed breast cancer patients were compared to an equal number of women without breast cancer. Based upon dietary surveys, and after adjusting for known breast cancer risk factors among these patient volunteers, the women who consumed the greatest amounts of "gim" seaweed were found to be *nearly 50 percent less likely* to develop breast cancer. Although case-control studies, such as this one, are of relatively low power, this interesting little study suggests that at least some types of seaweed might reduce the risk of developing breast cancer, and should be further studied using randomized, prospective clinical research trials [63].

Diabetes, Metformin (Glucophage) & Breast Cancer Prevention

As I have already briefly discussed earlier in this book, patients with diabetes are known to be at increased risk of developing certain types of cancer, including breast cancer [64]. Diabetes also appears to increase the risk of developing a recurrence of previously diagnosed cancers. Among other possible explanations, elevated levels of insulin are thought to act as a stimulus for cancer cells to grow and divide. Other diabetes-associated factors also appear to cause increased cancer cell proliferation, or growth, including insulin-like growth factor (IGF).

Metformin, also known as Glucophage, has become the most commonly prescribed oral medication for the treatment of diabetes. Previous laboratory and public health studies have suggested that metformin may also be able to suppress cancer cell growth (proliferation), and reduce the risk of death due to cancer. However, there has been very little direct evidence available to confirm these observations. Recently, though, in a retrospective clinical study from the M.D. Anderson Cancer Center, the medical records of 2,529 patients who received chemotherapy as initial treatment (neoadjuvant chemotherapy) for breast cancer, between 1990 and 2007, were reviewed [65]. This group of breast cancer patients included 68 diabetic patients who were taking metformin, 87 diabetic patients who were *not* taking metformin, and 2,374 nondiabetic patients. All

2,529 patients subsequently went on to have surgery for their breast cancers, and the researchers then assessed the response of each woman's breast cancer to their initial chemotherapy. The incidence of pathological complete response to neoadjuvant chemotherapy was then evaluated in each of the three groups of women involved in this clinical study. (A pathological complete response to chemotherapy occurs when the pathologist can no longer find any evidence of residual cancer after surgical removal of the original cancer site. This is an important finding, as a pathological complete response to neoadjuvant chemotherapy is generally associated with a better prognosis.)

In this study, the diabetic women who were taking metformin were found to have *3 times the rate* of pathological complete response to neoadjuvant chemotherapy when compared to the diabetic women who were not taking metformin (there was also a nonsignificant trend towards improved pathological complete response in the metformin group of diabetic women when compared to the nondiabetic women who, of course, were not taking metformin).

While the retrospective nature of this study, and the relatively small numbers of diabetic women included in the study, significantly limits the conclusions that can be drawn, these results are consistent with other previous research findings. Taken together, this data strongly suggests that metformin may be able to, at a minimum, counteract the proliferative effects of diabetes on breast cancer cells. These findings also raise the question of whether or not diabetic women who are diagnosed with breast cancer should be routinely placed on metformin as part of their overall cancer treatment program. Since this clinical study also detected a non-significant improvement in pathological complete response rates among diabetic women taking metformin, when compared to nondiabetic women, larger prospective clinical research studies may also help us to understand whether or not metformin might be clinically useful in treating breast cancer in women who do *not* have diabetes, as well.

Non-Steroidal Anti-Inflammatory Drugs & Breast Cancer Prevention

Anti-inflammatory drugs, collectively referred to as NSAIDs (nonsteroidal anti-inflammatory drugs), include the familiar medications aspirin, ibuprofen, naproxen, and Celebrex, among others. NSAIDS have previously been shown to reduce the incidence of precancerous polyps and cancers of the colon and rectum in high-risk patients. There is also some low-level data suggesting that these drugs might also decrease breast cancer risk as well [66].

The enormous Nurses' Health Study, which has recruited more than 121,000 women since its inception in 1976, has recently identified a significant reduction in the risk of breast cancer recurrence, and death due to breast cancer, in women previously diagnosed with breast cancer who regularly take aspirin. However, no decrease in the risk of developing a new breast cancer was identified in this huge ongoing prospective public health study. Therefore, this study did not identify any apparent cancer *prevention* effect associated with regular aspirin consumption [67].

Recent clinical research has not been very kind to *non-aspirin* NSAIDs, either. Recent large-scale prospective clinical research trials have clearly linked Celebrex, Vioxx, ibuprofen, and other *non-aspirin* NSAIDs with an *increased* risk of cardiovascular disease, heart attack, and other serious cardiovascular events. These unfavorable research findings have significantly cooled much of the previous enthusiasm for the routine use of *non-aspirin* NSAIDs as cancer prevention agents, except in patients who are known to be at very high risk of developing colorectal polyps and cancers.

Anti-Estrogen Medications & Breast Cancer Prevention

For women who are at especially high risk of developing breast cancer, including women with BRCA1 or BRCA2 gene mutations, the option of anti-estrogen (hormonal) therapy (i.e., breast cancer chemoprevention) may be considered.

Based upon landmark prospective breast cancer prevention trials, we know that high-risk women can cut their risk of developing breast cancer roughly in half by taking tamoxifen or raloxifene for 5 years. These medications belong to a class of drugs called SERMs (Selective Estrogen Receptor Modulators), and they work by blocking the estrogen receptors contained within both benign and malignant breast cells. This "antagonist" action of SERMs prevents the binding of estrogen to cellular estrogen receptors, thus shutting down estrogen's signal for these cells to grow and divide. However, as with most other medications, these drugs are associated with significant, and occasionally life-threatening, potential side effects. For example, tamoxifen is associated with a small but significant increase in the risk of developing uterine cancer, and so women taking this medication must be screened each year for uterine cancer. (On the other hand, however, both tamoxifen and raloxifene significantly decrease the risk of osteoporosis and hip fractures.) Women who are at high risk of developing breast cancer should carefully discuss their own individual health risk factors with an oncology physician before deciding to take a SERM as a breast cancer prevention measure.

Prophylactic Mastectomy & Breast Cancer Prevention

In some cases, surgery may also be considered for women who have an especially high lifetime risk of developing breast cancer. This is particularly the case for women who have been confirmed to carry one of the hereditary breast cancer gene mutations that I have previously discussed. Prophylactic bilateral mastectomy, or the surgical removal of both of a woman's breasts, is, admittedly, the most radical possible method of preventing breast cancer. However, for women with BRCA1 or BRCA2 gene mutations, prophylactic bilateral mastectomy is one option to consider in view of the very high lifetime risk of breast cancer associated with either of these gene mutations. As with the decision to take SERM medications (which is also a valid option for women with BRCA mutations), prophylactic mastectomy is an option that should be carefully considered, and then only after extensive consultations with oncology physicians and surgeons with expertise in this area. It should also be noted that bilateral prophylactic mastectomy yields a lifetime breast cancer risk reduction level of approximately 95 percent. As microscopic traces of breast cells are left behind after mastectomy, even this most radical of breast cancer prevention options is still not 100 percent protective against this disease in high-risk women (although it is as close to a 100 percent reduction in risk as can be attained). (Prophylactic surgical removal of both ovaries should also be considered in women with BRCA mutations, to prevent ovarian cancer.)

Summary of Breast Cancer Prevention Strategies

In summary, while not all breast cancers are preventable through modifications in lifestyle and diet, the cumulative epidemiological breast cancer data suggests that *at least 40 percent* of all breast cancer cases could be prevented simply by avoiding the use of hormone replacement therapy, limiting (or eliminating) alcohol consumption, avoiding obesity (especially during adulthood) and smoking, reducing meat and fat consumption, and by engaging in regular and moderate exercise [68]. As an added bonus, these very same breast cancer prevention lifestyle strategies will also significantly reduce your risk of other cancers, as well as reducing your risk of life-threatening cardiovascular disease at the same time.

Currently, with the possible exception of Vitamin D, there is no high-level research evidence of any significant breast cancer prevention effect associated with the use of vitamin supplements [69].

Finally, given that as many as 60 percent of new breast cancer cases may still not be preventable via lifestyle and dietary modifications, alone, women can still markedly reduce their lifetime risk of dying from breast cancer by adhering to established breast cancer screening guidelines, as I have outlined in this chapter. Currently, more than 90 percent of patients who are diagnosed with invasive breast cancer at the earliest detectable stage can anticipate being free of cancer recurrence 5 years later, and approximately 80 percent of women with early-stage breast cancer will remain disease-free 10 years after their diagnosis.

References

1. Cancer Facts & Figures 2009, The American Cancer Society.

2. Cancer Facts & Figures 2009, The American Cancer Society.

3. U.S. News & World Report, June 13, 2005.

4. Malone KE, et al. Prevalence and predictors of BRCA1 and BRCA2 mutations in a population-based study of breast cancer in white and black American women ages 35 to 64 years. *Cancer Research* 2006; 66:8297-8308.

5. John EM, et al. Prevalence of Pathogenic BRCA1 Mutation Carriers in 5 US Racial/Ethnic Groups. *Journal of the American Medical Association* 2008; 298:2869-2876.

6. Weitzel JN, et al. Limited Family Structure and BRCA Gene Mutation Status in Single Cases of Breast Cancer. Journal of the American Medical Association 2007; 297:2587-2595.

7. Rossouw JE, et al. Risks and benefits of estrogen plus progestin in healthy postmenopausal women: principal results From the Women's Health Initiative randomized controlled trial. *Journal of the American Medical Association* 2002; 288:321-333.

8. Reeves GK, et al. Cancer incidence and mortality in relation to body mass index in the Million Woman Study: cohort study. *British Medical Journal* 2007; 335:1134-1145]

9. Singletary SE. Rating the risk factors for breast cancer. *Annals of Surgery* 2003; 237:474–482.

10. Li Y, et al. Wine, liquor, beer and risk of breast cancer in a large population. *European Journal of Cancer* 2008 [Epub ahead of print].

11. Deandrea S, et al. Alcohol and breast cancer risk defined by estrogen and progesterone receptor status: a case-control study. *Cancer Epidemiology, Biomarkers & Prevention* 2008; 17:2025-2028.

12. Engeset D, et al. Dietary patterns and risk of cancer of various sites in the Norwegian European Prospective Investigation into Cancer and Nutrition cohort: the Norwegian Women and Cancer study. *European Journal of Cancer Prevention* 2009; 18:69-75.

13. Duffy CM, et al. Alcohol and folate intake and breast cancer risk in WHI Observational Study. *Breast Cancer Research & Treatment* 2008 [Epub ahead of print].

14. Mahoney MC, et al. Opportunities and Strategies for Breast Cancer Prevention Through Risk Reduction. *CA, A Cancer Journal for Clinicians* 2008; 58:347-371.

15. Cho E, et al. Red meat intake and risk of breast cancer among premenopausal women. *Archives of Internal Medicine* 2006; 166:2253–2259.

16. Taylor EF, et al. Meat consumption and risk of breast cancer in the UK Women's Cohort Study. *British Journal of Cancer* 2007; 96:1139–1146.

17. Kuper H, et al. Job strain and risk of breast cancer. *Epidemiology* 2007; 18:764-768'

18. Schernhammer ES, et al. Job stress and breast cancer risk: the nurses' health study. *American Journal of Epidemiology* 2004; 160:1079-1086.

19. Reynolds P. et al. Passive smoking and risk of breast cancer in the California teachers study. *Cancer Epidemiology, Biomarkers & Prevention* 2009; 18:3389-3398.

20. Lawrence G, et al. Population estimates of survival in women with screen-detected and symptomatic breast cancer taking account of

lead time and length bias. *Breast Cancer Research & Treatment* 2008 [Epub ahead of print].

21. Le-Petross HT, et al. Effectiveness of screening women at high risk for breast cancer with alternating mammography and MRI. (Presentation at the San Antonio Breast Cancer Symposium, December 2008.)

22. Ahn J, et al. Adiposity, adult weight change, and postmenopausal breast cancer risk. *Archives of Internal Medicine* 2007; 167:2091-2102.

23. Monninkhof EM, Elias SG, Vlems FA, et al. Physical activity and breast cancer: a systematic review. *Epidemiology* 2007; 18:137–157.

24. Schmidt ME, at al. Physical activity and postmenopausal breast cancer: effect modification by breast cancer subtypes and effective periods in life. *Cancer Epidemiology, Biomarkers & Prevention* 2008; 17:3402-3410.

25. World Cancer Research Fund and American Institute for Cancer Research. Food, Nutrition, Physical Activity, and the Prevention of Cancer: A Global Perspective 2007. Washington, DC: World Cancer Research Fund and American Institute for Cancer Research; 2007.

26. Peplonska B, et al. Adulthood lifetime physical activity and breast cancer. *Epidemiology* 2008; 19:226-246.

27. Maruti SS, et al. A prospective study of age-specific physical activity and premenopausal breast cancer. *Journal of the National Cancer Institute* 2008; 100:728-737.

28. Breast cancer and breastfeeding: collaborative reanalysis of individual data from 47 epidemiological studies in 30 countries, including 50,302 women with breast cancer and 96,973 women without the disease. *Lancet* 2002; 360:187–195.

29. Thiébaut AC, et al. Dietary fat and postmenopausal invasive breast cancer in the National Institutes of Health-AARP Diet and

Health Study cohort. *Journal of the National Cancer Institute* 2007; 99:451-462.

30. Wang J, et al. Dietary fat, cooking fat, and breast cancer risk in a multiethnic population. *Nutrition & Cancer* 2008; 60:492-504.

31. Velie E, et al. Dietary fat, fat subtypes, and breast cancer in post-menopausal women: a prospective cohort study. *Journal of the National Cancer Institute* 2000; 92:833-839.

32. Sieri S, et al. Dietary patterns and risk of breast cancer in the ORDET cohort. *Cancer Epidemiology, Biomarkers & Prevention* 2004; 13:567-572.

33. Thiébaut AC, et al. Dietary fat and postmenopausal invasive breast cancer in the National Institutes of Health-AARP Diet and Health Study cohort. *Journal of the National Cancer Institute* 2007; 99:451-462.

34. Wang J, et al. Dietary fat, cooking fat, and breast cancer risk in a multiethnic population. *Nutrition & Cancer* 2008; 60:492-504.

35. Pierce JP, et al. Influence of a diet very high in vegetables, fruit, and fiber and low in fat on prognosis following treatment for breast cancer: the Women's Healthy Eating and Living (WHEL) randomized trial. *Journal of the American Medical Association* 2007; 298:289–298.

36. LaVecchia C, Bosetti C. Diet and cancer risk in Mediterranean countries: open issues. *Public Health & Nutrition* 2006; 9:1077-1082.

37. Chlebowski RT, et al. Calcium Plus Vitamin D Supplementation and the Risk of Breast Cancer. *Journal of the National Cancer Institute* 2008; 100:1581-1591.

38. Shin MH, et al. Intake of dairy products, calcium, and vitamin D and risk of breast cancer. *Journal of the National Cancer Institute* 2002; 94:1301–1311.

39. Bertone-Johnson ER, et al. Plasma 25-hydroxyvitamin D and 1,25-dihydroxyvitamin D and risk of breast cancer. *Cancer Epidemiology, Biomarkers & Prevention* 2005; 14:1991–1997.

40. Crew KD, et al. Association between plasma 25-hydroxyvitamin D and breast cancer risk. *Cancer Prevention Research* 2009; 2:598-604.

41. Chen P, et al. Meta-analysis of vitamin D, calcium and the prevention of breast cancer. *Breast Cancer Research & Treatment* 2009; Oct 23. [Epub ahead of print].

42. Rejnmark L, et al. Reduced prediagnostic 25-hydroxyvitamin D levels in women with breast cancer: a nested case-control study. *Cancer Epidemiology, Biomarkers & Prevention* 2009; 18:2655-2660.

43. Zhang SM, et al. Effect of combined Folic Acid, Vitamin B6, and Vitamin B12 on Cancer Risk in Women. *Journal of the American Medical Association* 2008; 300; 2012-1021.

44. Trock BJ, et al. Meta-analysis of soy intake and breast cancer risk. *Journal of the National Cancer Institute* 2006; 98:459–471.

45. Warri A, et al. The role of early life genistein exposures in modifying breast cancer risk. *British Journal of Cancer* 2008; 98:1485-1493.

46. Wu AH, et al. Adolescent and adult soy intake and risk of breast cancer in Asian-Americans. *Carcinogenesis* 2002; 23:1491–1496.

47. Shu XO, et al. Soyfood intake during adolescence and subsequent risk of breast cancer among Chinese women. *Cancer Epidemiology Biomarkers & Prevention* 2001; 10:483–488.

48. Thanos J, et al. Adolescent dietary phytoestrogen intake and breast cancer risk (Canada). *Cancer Causes & Control* 2006; 17:1253–1261.

49. Suzuki Y, et al. Green tea and the risk of breast cancer: pooled analyses of two prospective studies in Japan. *British Journal of Cancer* 2004; 90:1361-1363.

50. Zhang M, et al. Green tea and the prevention of breast cancer: a case-control study in Southeast China. *Carcinogenesis* 2007; 28:1074-1078.

51. Seely D, et al. The effects of green tea consumption on incidence of breast cancer and recurrence of breast cancer: a systematic review and meta-analysis. *Integrative Cancer Therapies* 2005; 4:144-155.

52. Le Corre L. et al. Resveratrol and breast cancer chemoprevention: molecular mechanisms. *Molecular Nutrition & Food Research* 2005; 49:462-471.

53. Aziz MH, et al. Cancer chemoprevention by resveratrol: in vitro and in vivo studies and the underlying mechanisms (review). *International Journal of Oncology* 2003; 23:17-23.

54. Levi F, et al. Resveratrol and breast cancer risk. *European Journal of Cancer Prevention* 2005; 14:139-142.

55. Mehta R, et al. Breast cancer chemoprevention properties of pomegranate (Punica granatum) fruit extracts in a mouse mammary organ culture. *European Journal of Cancer Prevention* 2004; 13:345-348.

56. Fowke JH, et al. Urinary isothiocyanate levels, and human breast cancer. *Cancer Research* 2003; 63:3980-3986.

57. Butler LM, et al. A vegetable-fruit-soy dietary pattern protects against breast cancer among postmenopausal Singapore Chinese women. *American Journal of Clinical Nutrition* 2010' 91:1013-1019.

58. Bergman Jungeström M, et al. Flaxseed and its lignans inhibit estradiol-induced growth, angiogenesis, and secretion of vascular endothelial growth factor in human breast cancer xenografts in vivo. *Clinical Cancer Research* 2007; 13:1061-1067.

59. Ghosh-Choudhury T, et al. Fish oil targets PTEN to regulate NF-Kappa-B for downregulation of anti-apoptotic genes in breast tumor growth. *Breast Cancer Research & Treatment* 2008 [Published Online: 10/26/2008].

60. Kim J, et al. Fatty fish and fish omega-3 fatty acid intakes decrease the breast cancer risk: a case-control study. *BMC Cancer* 2009; 9:216.

61. Anand P, et al. Curcumin and cancer: an "old-age" disease with an "age-old" solution. *Cancer Letters* 2008; 267:133-164.

62. Lopez-Lazaro M. Anticancer and carcinogenic properties of curcumin: considerations for its clinical development as a cancer chemopreventive and chemotherapeutic agent. *Molecular Nutrition & Food Research* 2008; 52 (Suppl 1):S103-S127.

63. Yang YJ, et al. A case-control study on seaweed consumption and the risk of breast cancer. *British Journal of Nutrition* 2009 [Epub ahead of print].

64. Vigneri P, et al. Diabetes and cancer. *Endocrine-Related Cancer* 2009; 16:1103-1123.

65. Jiralerspong S, et al. Metformin and pathologic complete response to neoadjuvant chemotherapy in diabetic patients with breast cancer. *Journal of Clinical Oncology* 2009; 27:3297-3302.

66. Bahi T, et al. Breast cancer and use of nonsteroidal anti-inflammatory drugs: a meta-analysis. *Journal of the National Cancer Institute* 2008; 100:1439-1447.

67. Holmes MD, et al. Aspirin intake and survival after breast cancer. *Journal of Clinical Oncology* 2010; 28:1467-1472.

68. Sprague BL, et al. Proportion of invasive breast cancer attributable to risk factors modifiable after menopause. *American Journal of Epidemiology* 2008; 168:404-411.

69. Michels KB, et al. Diet and breast cancer: a review of the prospective observational studies. *Cancer* 2007; 109(12 Suppl):2712-2749.

CHAPTER 16

PROSTATE CANCER

Overview of Prostate Cancer

The prostate gland is a walnut-sized organ that wraps around the male urethra at the base of the bladder. Multiple ducts connect the prostate gland to the urethra to allow the prostatic secretions to be expelled into the urethra at the time of ejaculation. These prostatic secretions, which constitute about 20 percent of the volume of semen, help to create the optimal chemical environment for sperm to thrive and migrate within the female genital tract, thereby enhancing sperm function.

In many respects, prostate cancer is the male counterpart of breast cancer in women. As is also true with breast cancer in women, prostate cancer is the most common cancer that occurs in men (excluding minor skin cancers), and the second most common cause of cancer death among men. Prostate cancer accounts for 25 percent of all cancer diagnoses in men (similar to the percentage of breast cancer cases among all cancer cases diagnosed in women), and, according to the American Cancer Society, approximately 1 of every 6 American men will be diagnosed with prostate cancer at some point in their lifetimes, while 1 out of every 35 men will die of this disease. In 2009, an estimated 192,000 new cases of prostate cancer were diagnosed in the United States, and approximately 27,000 American men died of this disease in the same year [1].

As with the great majority of breast cancer cases, most prostate cancers are stimulated to grow and spread by sex hormones produced by the gonads (and, specifically, by testosterone and other androgens).

Risk Factors for Prostate Cancer

Gender, Age & Prostate Cancer Risk

As prostate cancer occurs only in men, male gender is the single most significant risk factor for this type of cancer. Like most types of cancer, prostate cancer becomes increasingly more common with advancing age. (The average age at diagnosis with prostate cancer is 70 years, and two-thirds of all prostate cancer cases occur in men over the age of 65 years.) Autopsy studies have also found that as many as *80 percent* of men who die during their 7th decade of life (from causes other than prostate cancer) already have previously undiagnosed prostate cancers [2].

Race, Ethnicity & Prostate Cancer Risk

Although the exact reasons are not well understood yet, prostate cancer is 1.5 to 2 times more common in African-American men when compared to Caucasian men.

Family History & Hereditary Prostate Cancer Syndromes

It has been estimated that 5 to 10 percent of all prostate cancer cases are inherited. However, among men who develop prostate cancer at an early age, as many as *30 to 40 percent* of such cancers may be due to inherited genetic factors [3]. Interestingly, many inherited cases of prostate cancer have been attributed to the same BRCA gene mutations (and BRCA2 mutations, in particular) that are more commonly associated with inherited breast and ovarian cancers in women [4].

Genetic factors are also thought to underlie the dramatically higher incidence of prostate cancer among certain ethnic groups throughout the world, as well, although the precise genes involved are not well understood at this time.

Obesity & Prostate Cancer Risk

Although the link between obesity and prostate cancer does not appear to be as strong as the link between obesity and breast cancer, there is, nonetheless, evidence that obesity may increase the risk of developing prostate cancer, and more aggressive prostate cancers in particular. In one large study, more than

10,000 patient volunteers in the prospective Prostate Cancer Prevention Trial were carefully evaluated. In this study, obese men were *29 percent more likely* to develop high-grade (i.e., more aggressive) prostate cancers when compared to non-obese men [5].

Alcohol & Other Dietary Prostate Cancer Risk Factors

As with obesity, the link between alcohol intake and prostate cancer risk does not appear to be as strong as the link between alcohol and breast cancer. However, there is, nonetheless, clinical research data suggesting that frequent alcohol intake may indeed increase the risk of prostate cancer [6]. In one large prospective prostate cancer prevention research study, nearly 11,000 men were followed for an average of 7 years. In this public health study, drinking alcohol every day, or nearly every day, was associated with *more than 2 times* the risk of developing prostate cancer when compared to men who drank more modestly and less frequently [7].

Inflammation & Prostate Cancer Risk

While there are likely multiple specific causes of prostate cancer, chronic inflammation (including chronic prostatitis) may play an important role in the development of this form of cancer (as with other types of cancer) [8]. For example, clinical studies have shown that bacterial colonization within the prostate gland (and associated chronic prostatic inflammation) is significantly more common in patients with prostate cancer when compared to patients without prostate cancer [9].

Agent Orange Exposure & Prostate Cancer Risk

Agent Orange exposure may be linked to an increased risk of prostate cancer among Vietnam War veterans who were exposed to this herbicide during the War. Using the Veteran Administration's clinical database, more than 13,000 veterans of the Vietnam War were assessed in a recent study. Approximately 6,200 of these veterans were identified as having been exposed to Agent Orange during the War, while another 6,900 veterans were considered to have been "unexposed." Using this large clinical database, the incidence of prostate cancer in both groups of male veterans was assessed. The presence or absence of additional known risk factors for prostate cancer were also evaluated in these 13,000 men, including age, race, smoking history, family history of cancer, presence or absence of obesity, prostate-specific antigen (PSA) levels, and prior use of finasteride (a medication used to treat enlargement of the prostate gland, and which has also been shown to decrease the risk of developing prostate cancer).

When the researchers analyzed the two groups of male veterans, they found that prostate cancer was *more than 2 times as common* among the men who had been exposed to Agent Orange during the Vietnam War. Not only was prostate cancer more common among the men who had been exposed to Agent Orange, but their prostate cancers also appeared to occur at a slightly earlier age (the average age at diagnosis was 60 years among the exposed veterans versus 62 years for the unexposed vets). Moreover, the microscopic appearance, or grade, of prostate cancers that developed in the men exposed to Agent Orange was much more worrisome (i.e., higher grade) when compared to the cancers that occurred in the unexposed men. Finally, the veterans who were exposed to Agent Orange, and who developed prostate cancer, were *more than 3 times* as likely to already have spread of their cancer outside of the prostate gland at the time of diagnosis when compared to the men who had not been exposed to Agent Orange. When the researchers evaluated all of the other known risks factors for prostate cancer present in these two groups of men, only a history of Agent Orange exposure seemed to explain the striking differences in the incidence and severity of prostate cancers that were observed in this research study.

While this was a retrospective study, which increases the risk of introducing bias into its conclusions, the results are nevertheless quite compelling, especially in view of the fact that the researchers eliminated the most common risk factors for prostate cancer as potential explanations for the differences in prostate cancer risk observed between these two groups of veterans [10].

Frequency of Ejaculation & Prostate Cancer Risk

There is clinical research evidence available to suggest that regular sexual activity, involving ejaculation, may decrease the risk of developing prostate cancer. In one very large prospective study, more than 29,000 men between the ages of 46 and 81 years were followed for an average of 8 years. These patient volunteers provided extensive sexual histories, including their frequency of masturbation and sexual intercourse. During the nearly 10-year course of this study, 1,449 of these men were diagnosed with prostate cancer. The results of this study revealed that ejaculating *21 or more times per month* was associated with a *33 percent reduction* in the risk of prostate cancer when compared to men who reported 4 to 7 ejaculations per month [11]. (Needless to say, the findings of this research study are always popular with male patients, and men are generally anxious to share these results with their sexual partners....)

Vasectomy & Prostate Cancer Risk

A frequent concern among men contemplating vasectomy is that this anti-fertility surgery may result in an increased risk of prostate cancer. However, recent clinical studies have strongly suggested that there is *no* clinically significant link between vasectomy and prostate cancer risk. For example, in one such study, more than 1,000 men recently diagnosed with prostate cancer were compared to 942 men without prostate cancer. All of these study volunteers were matched with each other in terms of age, race, and other important factors known to be related to prostate cancer risk. This study found absolutely *no* difference in the percentage of prior vasectomy among the men in each of these two groups. (In both groups of men, 36 percent had previously undergone vasectomy for the purpose of sterilization.) Moreover, the men who had undergone vasectomy at a young age also did *not* experience any increased risk of developing prostate cancer when compared to the men who had undergone vasectomy later in life (or when compared to the men who had never undergone vasectomy) [12].

Smoking & Prostate Cancer Risk

In a large meta-analysis study of 24 prospective public health studies, encompassing 21,579 prostate cancer patients, the risk of prostate cancer was found to be *increased* proportionally to the amount and duration of cigarette smoking. Moreover, heavy smokers were found to experience up to a *30 percent increase* in the risk of dying from prostate cancer when compared to non-smokers [13].

Screening for Prostate Cancer

The death rate due to prostate cancer began to decline in the early 1990s, at about the same time that prostate-specific antigen (PSA) testing became common in the United States. While few experts dispute that using the PSA test to screen for prostate cancer has dramatically improved our ability to diagnose this form of cancer at a much earlier stage, there continues to be a great deal of debate about whether or not the widespread use of PSA testing has actually played a direct role in reducing the death rate due to prostate cancer. (The clinical research data linking routine PSA testing with prostate cancer death rates has, to date, been contradictory, with some studies suggesting that routine PSA testing reduces the risk of dying of prostate cancer, while other studies have found no such relationship between PSA testing and prostate cancer death risk. Even among internationally renowned prostate cancer experts, there continues to be a great deal of disagreement regarding the potential benefits, if any, of routine PSA testing as a screening tool to detect prostate cancer.)

Much of the controversy regarding the potential value of PSA testing is related to the somewhat unique biology of prostate cancer when compared to other types of cancer. Most types of cancer, if left untreated, will continue to rapidly grow and spread, eventually leading to the death of their hosts. In many cases, however, prostate cancer remains a slow-growing disease that, in many men, causes few if any symptoms, and does not lead to death (particularly in elderly men). Therefore, while many men with potentially aggressive prostate cancers owe their lives to the PSA test that diagnosed their cancer at an early stage, many other men with slow-growing and non-life-threatening prostate cancers will undergo unnecessary and aggressive prostate cancer treatments because their cancers were, likewise, detected by a PSA test. Since most approved treatments for prostate cancer are associated with a significant risk of complications, many prostate cancer experts worry that too many men are undergoing essentially unnecessary treatment for indolent prostate cancers that might never have been otherwise been detected (and, hence, treated) without a PSA blood test. This concern regarding the potential "overtreatment" of prostate cancer is the primary reason why some experts have advocated against routine PSA testing as a prostate cancer screening tool.

Two randomized, prospective clinical trials, recently published in the prestigious *New England Journal of Medicine*, add further fuel to the ongoing debate regarding the routine use of PSA testing to screen for prostate cancer in otherwise healthy men:

The first clinical trial was performed in the United States, between 1993 and 2001. The Prostate, Lung, Colorectal, and Ovarian (PLCO) Screening Trial enrolled nearly 77,000 men, and divided them into two roughly equal groups. The first group was offered annual screening with PSA testing for a period of 6 years and annual digital rectal exams for 4 years. Among the men in this "screened group," 85 percent underwent the scheduled PSA testing and

86 percent underwent the scheduled digital rectal examinations. The second group was not offered PSA testing or digital rectal examinations. (Although, as some critics of this study have pointed out, more than half of the men in this "control" group still actually received PSA testing from their personal physicians during the course of this study, and nearly half of the men in this control group also reported receiving digital rectal examinations during the clinical study period, as well.)

After an average of almost 10 years of follow-up, 2,820 men in the "screened group" were diagnosed with prostate cancer, while 2,322 new cases of prostate cancer were diagnosed among the "unscreened group" of men. *Although there was a 22 percent increase noted in the incidence of prostate cancer among the "screened group" of men, when compared with those in the "unscreened group," the death rate due to prostate cancer did not statistically differ between the two groups of men.* Therefore, the authors of this study concluded that, while more cases of prostate cancer were detected among the group of men who underwent routine annual PSA testing and digital rectal examination, there was essentially no difference in the death rate between the men who were rigorously screened and those who were not, following 10 years of observation [14].

The second prospective clinical study was performed in Europe, and evaluated more than 162,000 men (between the ages of 55 and 69) from 7 European countries. As with the previous study, the men participating in this public health study were randomly divided into two groups. The first group underwent PSA testing approximately every 4 years, while the men in the second group (control group) did not undergo PSA testing at all. This very large cohort of men was followed for an average of 9 years, during which 8.2 percent of the men in the PSA-screened group were diagnosed with prostate cancer and 4.8 percent of the men in the unscreened-group were diagnosed with prostate cancer. Unlike the American study (above), however, this much larger European study found a small but significant *improvement in survival* among the men who were routinely screened with PSA testing, with an observed *20 percent reduction* in the *relative* risk of death due to prostate cancer among the men who had undergone routine PSA testing. At the same time, the *absolute* difference in the risk of dying of prostate cancer between the two groups of men was quite small (0.71 deaths per 1,000 men), which translates into the need to screen 1,410 men, and to invasively treat 48 men with prostate cancer, before one death from prostate cancer could be prevented. Therefore, the results of this very large prospective, randomized clinical research trial appeared to confirm the concerns of those experts who believe that while routine PSA testing may save some lives, it also subjects many more men to unnecessary treatments that expose these men to all of the risks of such treatment, but without any potential clinical benefit in terms of their prostate cancer [15].

In view of the relatively short duration of patient follow-up in both of these prostate cancer studies, their conclusions may be premature, as the majority of cases of prostate cancer are relatively slow-growing, and even patients with metastatic prostate cancer can live for many years while receiving hormonal therapy and other treatments. (Because the death rate from prostate cancer is typically very low during the first 10 years following diagnosis, some experts have already offered a "middle-ground" recommendation for routine PSA testing, suggesting that men who are not likely to live more than 10 years, due to other ailments, should not undergo routine PSA testing. Along the same lines, ·many experts also recommend that men over the age of 75 also not undergo routine PSA testing, as they are rather unlikely to die of prostate cancer if they should develop the disease at this stage of their lives.)

So, although the recent publication of these two very important prostate cancer screening trials has generated a great deal of discussion in both the lay and medical communities, they have not, in fact, appreciably altered the overall debate regarding the routine use of PSA testing (and routine clinical prostate examinations) as a screening tool for prostate cancer. Fundamentally, in my view, this debate will continue to rage on until we are able to accurately (and prospectively) identify those cases of prostate cancer that actually need to be treated, versus those cases that can be safely observed. At the present time, however, we simply cannot reliably determine which patients should undergo invasive treatments for prostate cancer and which patients can safely be offered only "watchful waiting," and this is really the crux of the dilemma surrounding the issue of routine PSA testing. This leaves men (and their physicians) to make their decisions regarding routine PSA testing against a backdrop of confusing and contradictory research data, unfortunately. Therefore, at the present time, if you are 50 years old or older (or if you are 40 years old, or older, and you are an African-American man, or you have a family history of prostate cancer), you should discuss the issue of PSA testing with your primary physician or your urologist before choosing to have a PSA blood test performed.

Prostate Cancer Prevention Strategies

Exercise & Prostate Cancer Prevention

Regular exercise has been shown by some research studies to reduce the risk of prostate cancer, while other studies have revealed no apparent association between regular exercise and prostate cancer risk. In one rather small study, 190 men who were scheduled to undergo prostate biopsy to rule-out cancer provided detailed information describing their frequency and duration of mild, moderate, and strenuous exercise in a typical week. All of these men then subsequently underwent biopsy of their prostate glands. After adjusting for differences in known prostate cancer risk factors among these men, the authors of this study determined that the men who undertook vigorous and frequent exercise (9 mets per week, or more) were *65 percent less likely* to develop prostate cancer. Moreover, among the men who exercised moderately and frequently (3 to 8.9 mets per week), but who still developed prostate cancer, there was a dramatic *decrease* in the incidence of high-grade (i.e., aggressive) prostate cancer [16]. While this is a relatively low-powered clinical study, it does at least suggest that regular, vigorous exercise may reduce prostate cancer risk.

For additional information on the role of exercise in prostate cancer prevention, please also review Chapter 11 (**Exercise & Cancer Prevention**) in this book.

Diet & Prostate Cancer Prevention

As previously discussed, dietary habits appear to play a powerful role in the risk of multiple types of cancers, including most cancers of the gastrointestinal tract, and cancers of the uterus, kidney, and breast. While the data linking prostate cancer risk with dietary fat intake is not as robust as for other types of cancer, there is at least some evidence that a high-fat diet may increase the risk of prostate cancer, as well.

In a dietary survey-based study of 512 men with prostate cancer and 838 men without prostate cancer, men who reported the highest level of fat intake were found to have *more than twice the risk* of developing prostate cancer when compared to men who consumed very low-fat diets. Interestingly, this study evaluated only men below the age of 60 and, therefore, included men who developed the onset of prostate cancer at a younger than usual age [17].

Another study, a small prospective dietary intervention study, randomized 18 men with newly diagnosed prostate cancer to either a typical high-fat Western diet (with 40 percent of calories derived from fat) or a low-fat, high-fiber, soy-supplemented diet for a period of 4 weeks. In this innovative little study, blood was collected from the men in both groups, after a period of fasting, and the serum from this blood was used to treat human prostate cancer cells growing in a laboratory culture dish. While the serum of the men in the Western diet group had no effect on the growth of cultured human prostate cancer cells, the serum of the men in the low-fat diet group significantly decreased the growth of the cultured prostate cancer cells. When the researchers studied the fat composition of the serum collected from the men on a low-fat diet, they found that the concentrations of omega-6 fatty acids (which have pro-inflammatory activity) were significantly *reduced*, and the concentrations of omega-3 fatty acids (which have anti-inflammatory activity) were significantly *increased* when compared to the serum from the men in the Western diet group. While this study certainly does not prove that a low-fat diet can prevent or treat prostate cancer, it does at least suggest a biological mechanism whereby a low-fat diet *might* reduce the risk of developing prostate cancer. Moreover, there is no doubt but that a low-fat diet also reduces the risk of other types of cancer and cardiovascular disease [18]. (There is also additional laboratory research data available suggesting that a low-fat diet may reduce the growth, or proliferation, of human prostate cancer cells, which is discussed in the **Flaxseed & Prostate Cancer Prevention** section, later in this chapter.)

As I have discussed in the general section on diet and cancer risk, earlier in this book, there are numerous epidemiological studies that have linked a diet rich in fresh fruits and vegetables with an overall decreased risk of cancer and cancer-associated death. The data regarding prostate cancer risk and the consumption of fruits and vegetables, specifically, has been rather inconsistent. However, in a recent prospective clinical study, the very large Prostate, Lung, Colorectal and Ovarian Cancer Screening Trial, more than 29,000 men participated, and were followed for more than 4 years, on average. During this study period, 1,338 of these men were newly diagnosed with prostate cancer. Based upon detailed dietary surveys, the researchers conducting this study found no significant association between fruit and vegetable intake, in general, and the risk of prostate cancer. However, the *relative* risk of developing *advanced stages* of prostate cancer (stages III and IV) was *59 percent lower* among the men who reported consistently high intakes of fresh fruits and vegetables. Upon further analysis, the frequent consumption of cruciferous vegetables, and broccoli and cauliflower in particular, was determined to be the most important single dietary factor in the observed decrease in the incidence of advanced prostate cancers [19].

Once again, the data supporting a link between fresh fruit and vegetable consumption and prostate cancer risk is inconsistent, but there is ample and convincing data that a low-fat, high-fiber diet that is rich in highly-colored fresh fruits and vegetables (and cruciferous vegetables, in particular) is associated with a significantly reduced overall risk of cancer, cancer-associated mortality, cardiovascular disease, and mortality due to cardiovascular disease.

Antioxidant Vitamins, Dietary Supplements & Prostate Cancer Prevention

As with almost all published research looking at the prevention of cancer through dietary and nutritional supplements, there is data suggesting that certain nutrients may potentially reduce the risk of prostate cancer. As I have emphasized throughout this book, however, the majority of this type of research has been in the form of relatively low-powered public health studies, and from laboratory research using cancer cells growing in cell cultures, or immunodeficient mice implanted with human cancer cells. Although higher powered prospective randomized, placebo-controlled human research trials provide "gold standard" Level 1 research data, such studies are enormously expensive and difficult to undertake. However, when high quality prospective, randomized, blinded, placebo-controlled cancer prevention studies *are* performed to validate the findings of lower level research studies, the results are often quite disappointing. Such is the case with Vitamin E and selenium, both of which were previously identified as potential prostate cancer prevention agents in multiple low-powered research studies.

Based upon low-level epidemiology studies, Vitamin E and selenium appeared to be promising candidates as prostate cancer prevention agents. In fact, because multiple public health studies appeared to link these nutrients to a decreased risk of prostate cancer, a large prospective, randomized, blinded, placebo-controlled multi-institutional clinical study was recently performed. The Selenium and Vitamin E Cancer Prevention Trial (SELECT) enrolled more than 35,000 middle-aged and elderly men at 427 different medical centers in the United States, Canada, and Puerto Rico. These patient volunteers were randomized into one of 4 different intervention groups: selenium plus a placebo (sugar) pill, Vitamin E plus a placebo pill, Vitamin E and selenium pills, or 2 placebo pills. *After more than 5 years of follow-up, on average, there was no observed reduction in the risk of prostate cancer, or any other cancer, in any of the 3 groups of men who received selenium and/or Vitamin E* (in fact, there was a statistically nonsignificant *increase* in the incidence of prostate cancer among the group of men who had been randomly assigned to receive only Vitamin E) [20].

Another large prospective, randomized, placebo-controlled clinical study recruited nearly 15,000 healthy male physicians, and evaluated the effects of both Vitamin E and Vitamin C supplements (versus identical-appearing placebo sugar pills) on cancer risk. Following an average follow-up duration of 8 years, this Harvard Medical School study determined that *Vitamin C and Vitamin E supplements had absolutely no impact on the incidence of prostate cancer, or any other type of cancer* [21].

Lycopene & Prostate Cancer Prevention

Lycopene, like selenium and Vitamin E, has been suggested to have anti-cancer properties in the prostate gland, based upon previous laboratory and epidemiological research. However, more recently, this member of the Vitamin A family has not fared so well in human prostate cancer studies.

A prospective clinical study of 997 middle-aged men, with an average follow-up of nearly 13 years, evaluated the blood levels of lycopene versus the incidence of cancer. While higher levels of lycopene in the blood appeared to be associated with a *lower overall risk of cancer*, high levels of lycopene did *not* appear to offer any protection against prostate cancer, specifically [22].

In another prospective prostate cancer study, 17 men with advanced prostate cancer were given daily supplements of lycopene, and their response to this supplementation was then followed for an average of 20 months. The researchers conducting this very small pilot study found *no* evidence of any clinical improvement in the progression of prostate cancer in these 17 men associated with lycopene supplements, and no significant decreases in prostate-specific antigen (PSA) levels in these patients were noted, either [23].

Soy Isoflavones (Genistein), Resveratrol & Prostate Cancer Prevention

Soy-derived isoflavones are phytoestrogens that have weak estrogen-like activity in some organs and tissues of the human body. For this reason, soy isoflavones have been studied as potential prostate cancer prevention agents.

In addition to my previous general discussion of soy isoflavones as potential prostate cancer prevention agents, earlier in this book, there is additional research data linking soy isoflavones to a potential decrease in prostate cancer risk.

In an interesting laboratory animal study, using a rat model of prostate cancer, rats were fed either genistein (the predominant isoflavone in soybeans), or resveratrol, or a combination of both nutritional supplements. This study determined that rats fed high-dose genistein or resveratrol, or both, were significantly *less likely* to develop prostate cancer when compared to rats that received neither of these supplements, *and* also when compared to rats that received only low doses of both genistein and resveratrol. While animal models for disease prevention and treatment often fail to predict the effects of the same treatments in humans, this elegant laboratory study does suggest at least the *possibility* that soy isoflavones, and genistein in particular, may be able to reduce the risk of prostate cancer in humans (and, perhaps, resveratrol as well) [24].

In yet another very elegant and intriguing laboratory research study, the deactivation of a tumor suppressor gene known as B-Cell Translocation Gene 3 was identified in human prostate cancer cells. This gene, when functioning normally, is known to inhibit the development of cancer within the prostate gland. After discovering that this tumor suppressor gene was deactivated (by "demethylation" of this gene) in prostate cancer cells, the scientists then treated these same cancer cells with varying concentrations of soy-derived genistein. Higher concentrations of genistein were found to "reactivate" this prostate cancer tumor suppressor gene, raising the possibility that genistein may be able to reverse at least one of the genetic abnormalities that are thought to give rise to prostate cancer in humans [25].

In a meta-analysis of 13 previously published epidemiology studies, high levels of soy-food intake was associated with a *31 percent decrease* in the risk of prostate cancer. Tofu appeared to provide the greatest protection against prostate cancer, while soy milk appeared to have *no effect* on prostate cancer risk in this study [26].

A prospective, early-phase, clinical pilot study from Canada evaluated the effects of a soy beverage ("soy milk") on the progression of recurrent prostate cancer in 29 men following radiation therapy for their cancers. This study was not a placebo-controlled randomized study, however, this small phase II clinical study prospectively followed these patient volunteers for 6 months. During the course of this small study, serial measurements of blood levels of prostate-specific antigen (PSA) were performed (PSA is the primary prostate tumor marker that is measured both to detect early prostate cancer and to identify recurrences of this type of cancer.) The time interval during which the level of PSA in the blood doubles is an important indicator of the rate of progression of recurrent prostate cancer. In this small prospective clinical pilot study, the consumption of approximately 500 milliliters (ml) of soy beverage per day, for 6 months, was associated with an actual *decline in PSA levels* in 4 (14 percent) of these patient volunteers, while another 8 (28 percent) of these recurrent prostate cancer patients experienced a *greater than 100 percent increase in their PSA doubling times*. However, another 5 patients (17 percent) experienced a *50 percent or greater decrease in their PSA doubling times* during the 6 month duration of this study, which was an unfavorable development. Thus, during the brief duration of this intriguing but small pilot study, 42 percent of men with early recurrence of their prostate cancer experienced either a decrease in the biochemical extent of their recurrent cancers or a significant biochemical slowing of the progression of their recurrent disease.

Whether or not longer durations of soy intake will be able to sustain the favorable results noted in this study is not clear at this time. More importantly, whether or not these observed favorable effects of daily soy intake on PSA levels and PSA doubling times will actually translate into prolonged survival (or not) is also unknown at this time. It will require several larger and longer-term randomized, placebo-controlled, blinded, prospective clinical trials of soy foods and soy isoflavone supplements to answer these critical questions (several of which are already underway). Meanwhile, the overall safety profile for moderate amounts of soy intake in men appears to be quite favorable, and so many prostate cancer experts are cautiously recommending soy-derived foods for men with prostate cancer, and for men who are at an increased risk of developing prostate cancer, pending the completion of these larger prostate cancer research studies [27].

Meanwhile, multiple clinical research studies carried out in Asia and in the West have also suggested that prostate cancer risk *may* be decreased by a diet rich in soy isoflavones [28, 29]. One particularly intriguing prospective clinical study from Australia randomized 29 men with prostate cancer to one of three groups. One group was randomized to receive bread enriched with soy isoflavones in their daily diet, while a second group received bread enriched with both soy isoflavones and linseed oil (both of which are rich in phytoestrogens). The third group, which served as this study's control group, received wheat bread that was identical in appearance to the bread received by the other two groups of men, but which contained only low levels of naturally-occurring phytoestrogens, and no added phytoestrogen supplements. All 29 of these male prostate cancer patient volunteers had their blood tested for prostate-specific antigen (PSA), a marker of prostate cancer activity, at the beginning of the study and again at the end of the study. The men who consumed the wheat bread *without* added phytoestrogens experienced a *13 percent decline* in their PSA levels during the course of this study, while the men who were randomized to receive the phytoestrogen-enriched bread experienced a *very significant 40 percent decline* in PSA levels. While this very small, brief-duration, prospective clinical study cannot definitively prove that phytoestrogens are able to prevent prostate cancer (or shrink existing prostate cancers), its finding that soy isoflavone dietary supplementation results in a significant decrease in PSA levels at least suggests that dietary soy phytoestrogens *may* have clinically significant biological activity against prostate cancer in humans [30].

Phytosterols & Prostate Cancer Prevention

Phytosterols are known to reduce the concentration of LDL (the "bad cholesterol") in the blood. Bark extracts from the African plum tree are rich in phytosterols, and have been used, for many years, in Europe for the treatment of benign prostate disorders, including the enlargement of the prostate gland that occurs with aging (benign prostatic hypertrophy, or BPH).

While there is very little human research data available regarding possible anti-cancer properties associated with phytosterols, there is an increasing amount of laboratory research data available. One such study investigated the effects of phytosterols extracted from the bark of the African plum tree (*Pygeum africanum*) on cultured human prostate cancer cells, and found that the growth and survival of these cancer cells were significantly inhibited by these phytosterols. Mice that are prone to developing prostate cancer were also fed African plum tree bark extract, and only *35 percent* of these mice developed prostate cancer, while *63 percent* of the mice that did *not* receive *Pygeum africanum* bark extract developed prostate cancer during the course of this study [31]. (Once again, however, it must be stated that the findings observed in animal studies often do not translate directly to humans when identical treatments are tested in randomized, prospective, placebo-controlled clinical trials.)

Therefore, there *may* be a role for plant-derived phytosterols in prostate cancer prevention.

Flaxseed & Prostate Cancer Prevention

There is some interesting prospective clinical research data suggesting that flaxseed supplements may have significant anti-cancer effects against prostate cancer. In one important prospective clinical trial, 161 men newly diagnosed with prostate cancer were randomized into one of four intervention groups. The control group of men continued with their usual diets. A second group of men were placed on a low-fat diet (less than 20 percent of daily caloric intake in the form of fat) *without* flaxseed supplementation. The third group of men was placed on flaxseed supplementation (30 grams per day), but were allowed to continue with their usual diets. Finally, the fourth group of men received 30 grams of flaxseed supplementation per day *in addition to* a low-fat diet.

Following prostate cancer surgery, the tumors of these men were evaluated for a protein known as Ki-67, which is a marker of active tumor growth (proliferation). This study revealed that, when compared to the control group, the men who were placed on a low-fat diet had *lower* levels of Ki-67 in their prostate cancer tumors, and the men who received flaxseed supplements, along with their regular diets, had *even less* Ki-67 protein in their tumors. Finally, the men who were placed on *both flaxseed supplements and a low-fat diet* had the *lowest amount* of Ki-67 protein in their tumors, among all four groups of men [32]. While this study did not address the clinical outcomes of these men as a result of flaxseed supplementation, these results, nonetheless, suggest that *both a low-fat diet and flaxseed supplementation* are associated with significant anti-cancer effects in men with prostate cancer. (Once again, a long-term prospective, randomized, placebo-controlled clinical research trial must be performed to definitively assess flaxseed as a prostate cancer prevention agent, although data from studies such as this small pilot study are suggestive of such an effect.)

Cruciferous Vegetables (Sulforaphane) & Prostate Cancer Prevention

While diet-based studies have tended not to show a consistent benefit associated with increased fruit and vegetable intake, in general, in the prevention of prostate cancer, there is some data available to suggest that cruciferous vegetable intake, specifically, may in fact reduce the risk of this common type of cancer (and as suggested by a clinical study that I reviewed in the previous **Diet & Prostate Cancer Prevention** section). In fact two different case-control studies have identified a surprisingly similar degree of prostate cancer risk reduction among men who regularly consume cruciferous vegetables.

The first case-control study enrolled 1,230 adult men under the age of 65 in the United States (628 men with newly diagnosed prostate cancer and 602 age-matched men without prostate cancer). All of these men completed detailed dietary surveys, and the resulting data was analyzed. No apparent association between fruit intake and prostate cancer risk was identified. However, three or more servings of cruciferous vegetables per week (when compared to less than one serving per week) was associated with a *41 percent reduction in the risk of developing prostate cancer* in this group of 1,230 adult men. As I have previously mentioned, case-control epidemiological studies, such as this one, provide much less powerful data than prospective, randomized, controlled clinical trials. However, this study does at least suggest that the frequent consumption of cruciferous vegetables may be associated with a significantly decreased risk of developing prostate cancer [33].

Additional research by my former colleagues at the University of Hawaii's Cancer Research Center *also* suggests that increased cruciferous vegetable intake may decrease the risk of prostate cancer. In this multi-center case-control study, 1,619 African-American, Caucasian, Japanese and Chinese men with recently diagnosed prostate cancer were evaluated, along with a control group of 1,619 men of similar age and ethnicity who did not have prostate cancer. Dietary surveys were completed by all of these male volunteers, and blood samples were also taken from these men to assess prostate-specific antigen (PSA) levels. This study found that an increased intake of beans (including soybeans) was associated with a *38 percent reduction* in the risk of developing prostate cancer. Frequent consumption of yellow-orange vegetables and cruciferous vegetables also appeared to reduce prostate cancer risk by *33 percent* and *39 percent*, respectively [34]. These beneficial effects of diet on prostate cancer risk appeared to be present among all of these men, regardless of ethnicity. (An increased intake of tomatoes and fruits did not appear to reduce prostate cancer risk, however.)

Vitamin D & Prostate Cancer Prevention

I have already extensively discussed Vitamin D, earlier in this book, as a potential cancer prevention agent for other types of cancer (and, most notably, for colorectal cancer). The data linking Vitamin D with a decreased risk of prostate cancer has not been consistent (a very common reality in cancer prevention research, unfortunately). For example, a large prospective clinical research study that measured Vitamin D levels in the blood of both prostate cancer patients and in age-matched men without prostate cancer not only failed to find an association between high levels of Vitamin D in the blood and prostate cancer risk, but also identified a statistically non-significant trend towards *more aggressive* prostate tumors among men with very high levels of Vitamin D in their blood. However, although the findings of this study suggest that very high levels of Vitamin D in the blood of patients already diagnosed with prostate cancer *might* be associated with more aggressive tumors, the correlation between blood levels of Vitamin D and tumor aggressiveness was not uniform, suggesting that this observation was not definitively proven by the data derived from this study. Another limitation of this particular study is that Vitamin D levels in the blood were only measured a single time during the course of this study (at the beginning of the study). It is, therefore, not possible to know whether or not Vitamin D levels might have fluctuated considerably during the period of several years while this study was being carried out [35].

On the other hand, in a small pilot clinical study, 15 patients with recurrent prostate cancer were administered 2,000 IU of Vitamin D per day. In 9 of these patients with advanced, treatment-refractory prostate cancer, the prostate cancer marker PSA either *declined or remained stable* for as long as 21 months, suggesting a potentially significant anti-cancer effect by higher doses of Vitamin D [36]. (Moreover, the time required for PSA levels to double in value was *significantly increased in 14 of these 15 patients* after the Vitamin D supplements were initiated.)

Thus, the role of vitamin D, if any, as a prostate cancer prevention agent is not well understood at this time. (At the present time, Harvard Medical School is conducting a prospective Vitamin D prostate cancer prevention trial, and this clinical trial is currently recruiting healthy African-American men.)

Green Tea & Prostate Cancer Prevention

Green tea, that mysterious and ancient drink from the Far East, has long been lauded as a health tonic and disease prevention agent. While there is some data suggesting that the catechins contained in green tea (as discussed earlier in this book) may decrease the risk of certain cancers, the data for green tea as a prostate cancer prevention agent has been very inconsistent, to date.

In a very large prospective study of nearly 20,000 Japanese men, the consumption of 5 or more cups of green tea (versus less than 1 cup per day) was *not* associated with any apparent decrease in the incidence of prostate cancer [37]. However, an even larger Japanese study came to a somewhat different conclusion. The prospective Japan Public Health Center-based Prospective Study included nearly 50,000 men between the ages of 40 and 69 years. This study determined that drinking 5 or more cups of green tea per day (versus less than 1 cup per day) *was associated with a 48 percent decrease in the risk of developing advanced prostate cancer. At the same time, there appeared to be no decrease in the incidence of early-stage prostate cancer among the men who consumed the most green tea* [38].

Unfortunately, the disparate findings of these two very large prospective Japanese epidemiogical studies cannot resolve the debate regarding green tea's potential effects on prostate cancer risk. Additionally, the incidence of prostate cancer in Japan is much lower than in the United States, and throughout much of Europe, suggesting potential environmental or/and genetic differences in prostate cancer biology among these different populations of men. Therefore, the findings from these Japanese studies may or may not be directly applicable to populations outside of East Asia.

Before one entirely gives up on green tea as a potential prostate cancer prevention agent, however, there is some interesting clinical data from the United States linking high-dose green tea polyphenols with an anti-cancer effect in men with prostate cancer.

In a small pilot study, 26 men with newly diagnosed prostate cancer took daily supplements of green tea polyphenols while they were awaiting prostate cancer surgery (1.3 grams of polyphenols per day). At both the beginning and the end of this short-term study, blood was drawn to assess for biochemical markers associated with the stage and extent of prostate cancer (this clinical study continued up until the day of surgery for these patient volunteers).

Prostate-specific antigen (PSA), which is uniquely secreted by both normal and malignant prostate gland cells, is the most commonly used blood marker for prostate cancer. PSA levels in the blood rise as prostate cancer progresses. When prostate cancer is successfully treated, PSA levels often become almost undetectable. (On the other hand, rising PSA levels following previous prostate cancer treatment almost always signify cancer recurrence.) Other important tumor-associated factors include vascular endothelial growth factor

(VEGF) and hepatocyte growth factor (HGF). These proteins are known to stimulate the growth and spread of many types of cancer, including prostate cancer. Other known adverse tumor growth factors include insulin-like growth factor (IGF), and IGF binding protein. *All* of these tumor growth factors were measured in the blood samples collected from these 26 men, both at the beginning of this brief study and at its conclusion.

Additionally, cancer-associated fibroblast cells, which are associated with multiple different types of cancer, including prostate cancer, and which are thought to secrete proteins that directly and indirectly increase tumor growth, were cultured in laboratory dishes in this study. These cancer-associated fibroblasts were then treated with green tea polyphenols. Changes in tumor-stimulating proteins from these prostate cancer-associated fibroblasts cells were then measured following green tea polyphenol treatment.

When all of the data was analyzed, some tantalizing results were discovered. Blood levels of PSA, VEGF, HGF, IGF and IGF binding protein were *all significantly decreased* following a *brief* period of dietary supplementation with green tea polyphenols. Additionally, VEGF and HGF secretion by prostate cancer-associated fibroblasts significantly decreased, as well, following treatment of these cultured cells with green tea polyphenols.

While this brief and small pilot study does not provide any direct proof that dietary supplementation with green tea polyphenols can prevent prostate cancer, or that they can significantly improve survival in patients already diagnosed with prostate cancer, it does offer indirect evidence (based upon a decrease in prostate cancer-associated tumor markers) that green tea polyphenols may be able to inhibit prostate cancer cell growth, and not only in cancer cells growing in a laboratory culture dish, but also in living, breathing human patients with prostate cancer [39].

As green tea is well-tolerated by most healthy adults, there is little downside to including this age-old drink as part of a cancer-prevention and cardiovascular disease-prevention lifestyle. Meanwhile, the obvious next step is to conduct several large, long-term, prospective, randomized, placebo-controlled clinical research trials to put the findings of this small but intriguing pilot study to the test. Fortunately, there are several such clinical trials already underway.

Pomegranate Juice & Prostate Cancer Prevention

Pomegranate juice extract, which is rich in both tannins and phenolic acids, has recently been studied as a potential prostate cancer prevention agent. For example, laboratory research with human prostate cancer cells has shown that pomegranate juice extract can inhibit prostate cancer cell growth, including aggressive prostate cancer cells that have become resistant to hormone-blocking medications [40].

In an early-phase clinical trial, 46 prostate cancer patients with rising prostate-specific antigen (PSA) levels after either surgery or radiation treatment were asked to drink 8 ounces of pomegranate juice per day. Prior to beginning this study, the average time interval during which the serum PSA level doubled in value (a marker of recurrent prostate cancer growth) in these men was 15 months. Once these men began drinking pomegranate juice on a daily basis, their average *PSA doubling time increased, very significantly, to 54 months*, suggesting a very potent clinical effect against prostate cancer cells by pomegranate juice. The researchers also collected serum from the blood of these patient volunteers, both before and after starting pomegranate juice treatment, and used this serum to treat human prostate cancer cells growing in a culture dish. In comparing the effects of "pre-treatment" serum versus "post-treatment" serum on these cell cultures, the scientists found that the serum collected *after* the onset of pomegranate juice treatment *decreased prostate cancer cell growth by 12 percent, and increased cancer cell death by 17 percent*. Taken together, the findings of this study strongly suggest that pomegranate juice is not only active against prostate cancer cells growing in a laboratory dish, but also against prostate cancer cells growing in humans with recurrent prostate cancer [41].

In another laboratory study, mice bred with defective immune systems were injected with human prostate cancer cells. Among the mice that were fed pomegranate juice, the growth of the implanted prostate cancer tumors were significantly *inhibited*, and blood levels of prostate-specific antigen (PSA) simultaneously *dropped* significantly, as well [42]. (Of course, it must be mentioned, once again, that what works in mice does not always work in humans, unfortunately.)

Most prostate cancers are sensitive to testosterone-blocking drugs, initially. However, over time, many prostate cancers subsequently become resistant to these hormone-blocking drugs. In a laboratory study, performed at the University of California-Los Angeles (UCLA), human prostate cancer cells growing in cell cultures were treated with pomegranate juice extract, which directly inhibited the growth of these cancer cells. In the second part of this study, immunodeficient mice were injected with human prostate cancer cells. Among the mice that were fed pomegranate juice, the prostate cancer tumors appeared to retain their sensitivity to hormone-blocking therapy, whereas the tumors of mice that did not receive pomegranate juice extract eventually became resistant to hormone-blocking therapy [43]. (This study is potentially clinically important, because it suggests that pomegranate juice might be able to prevent, or at least delay, the development of aggressive hormone-resistant tumors in men with prostate cancer.)

Lupeol & Prostate Cancer Prevention

Lupeol is naturally abundant in mangoes, and is also found in strawberries, red grapes, figs, olives, tomatoes, peppers, and cucumbers. In addition to its anti-inflammatory properties, lupeol has been shown, in laboratory research, to inhibit several different biological pathways necessary for cancer cell growth and survival. Prostate cancer cells may also be susceptible to inhibition by lupeol.

In one laboratory study, lupeol was found to directly *inhibit* multiple specific biological pathways related to prostate cancer cell growth and survival [44].

Statin Drugs & Prostate Cancer Prevention

There is some evidence that cholesterol-lowering statin drugs *might* reduce the risk of prostate cancer, including a study in Finland that evaluated more than 23,000 men between 1996 and 2004. In this study, statin use was associated with a *24 percent reduction* in the risk of developing prostate cancer. Moreover, longer durations of statin medication therapy were associated with an *even lower* level of prostate cancer risk [45]. Unfortunately, as previously discussed, the data regarding statin drugs as cancer prevention agents is quite contradictory.

Hormone-Blocking Medications & Prostate Cancer Prevention

Because most prostate cancers, like breast cancer, are fueled by sex hormones, the prevention of prostate cancer through the use of hormone-blocking medications is an attractive potential strategy.

Two medications, finasteride (Proscar) and dutasteride (Avodart), are FDA-approved to treat the benign enlargement of the prostate that commonly occurs with increasing age (also known as benign prostatic hypertrophy, or BPH). Both of these medications have recently been evaluated in prospective, randomized, placebo-controlled clinical research trials as potential prostate cancer prevention agents. Finasteride and dutasteride are 5-alpha-reductase inhibitors, and function by blocking the conversion of testosterone into dihydrotestosterone by this enzyme, which is the biologically active male sex hormone within the prostate gland. Finasteride inhibits one of the two known forms of 5-alpha-reductase, while dutasteride (Avodart) inhibits both forms.

Finasteride (Proscar) was evaluated in the Prostate Cancer Prevention Trial, which enrolled nearly 19,000 men (55 years of age and older) who were without any clinical evidence of prostate cancer at the time they entered the study. These men were randomly assigned to receive either finasteride or an identical placebo pill, and the entire cohort of men was then followed for a period of 7 years. After 7 years of follow-up, 18 percent of the men who had been secretly randomized to receive finasteride were diagnosed with prostate cancer, while 24 percent of the men who had received the placebo pill (unknown to them at the time) developed prostate cancer. Thus, taking finasteride for 7 years was associated with a *25 percent reduction* in the *relative* risk of prostate cancer during the rather brief course of this clinical study. However, a potentially significant downside was also observed in this study, as the men who received finasteride, *and* who still went on to develop prostate cancer, tended to have more aggressive tumors when compared to the men in the placebo group (*37 percent versus 22 percent*, respectively). Moreover, and not surprisingly, since finasteride blocks the formation of the active metabolite of testosterone, sexual dysfunction and breast enlargement were more common among the men taking finasteride when compared to the men in the placebo group [46].

Following the intriguing results with finasteride (Proscar) in the Prostate Cancer Prevention Trial, there has been a great deal of anticipation building for results of the comparable dutasteride (Avodart) prostate cancer prevention trial. Fortuitously, as I was editing the final manuscript of this book, the preliminary results from this prospective, randomized, placebo-controlled, double-blind clinical trial were published in the *New England Journal of Medicine*. This study lasted for 4 years, and included 6,729 men at high risk of developing prostate cancer. These men, all of whom were between 50 and 75 years of age, were secretly randomized to receive either 0.5 mg of dutasteride (Avodart) per day or an identical placebo pill. As part of this research study's protocol, all of these men underwent needle biopsies of their prostate glands at 2 years and 4 years after entering the study. By the end of the study, 20 percent of the men who had received dutasteride (Avodart) had developed prostate cancer, while 25 percent of the men in the placebo (control) group were diagnosed with prostate cancer. Thus, as was noted in the Proscar study, there was an observed *25 percent decrease* in the *relative* risk of prostate cancer among the group of men that was randomized to receive dutasteride (Avodart) for 4 years (and a *5 percent absolute reduction* in prostate cancer risk with Avodart). As was also observed in the finasteride (Proscar) study, however, there was a higher incidence of more aggressive (i.e., higher grade) tumors observed among the men who took dutasteride (Avodart) when compared to the men in the placebo group, although only a very small number of these aggressive looking tumors were identified in either group of men. Finally, as expected, the symptoms of benign prostatic hypertrophy (BPH), including difficulties in passing urine, were much improved among the men randomized to take dutasteride (Avodart) [47].

Because it is still too soon to determine whether or not finasteride or dutasteride actually save lives, there is no consensus at this time, among most prostate cancer experts, regarding the routine use of these hormone-blocking agents as prostate cancer prevention agents.

References

1. Cancer Facts & Figures 2009, The American Cancer Society.

2. Breslow N; et al. Latent carcinoma of prostate at autopsy in seven areas. The International Agency for Research on Cancer, Lyons, France. *International Journal of Cancer* 1977; 20:680–688.

3. Bratt O. Hereditary prostate cancer: clinical aspects. *Journal of Urology* 2002; 168:906-913.

4. Kirchhoff T, et al. BRCA mutations and risk of prostate cancer in Ashkenazi Jews. *Clinical Cancer Research* 2004; 10:2918-2921.

5. Gong Z, et al. Obesity, diabetes, and risk of prostate cancer: results from the Prostate Cancer Prevention Trial. *Cancer, Epidemiology, Biomarkers & Prevention* 2006; 15:1977-1983.

6. Benedetti A, et al. Lifetime consumption of alcoholic beverages and risk of 13 types of cancer in men: results from a case-control study in Montreal. *Cancer Detection & Prevention* 2009; 32:352-362.

7. Gong Z, et al. Alcohol consumption, finasteride, and prostate cancer risk: results from the Prostate Cancer Prevention Trial. *Cancer* 2009; 115:3661-3669.

8. Nelson WG, et al. The role of inflammation in the pathogenesis of prostate cancer. *Journal of Urology* 2004; 172:S6-S11.

9. Sciarra A, et al. Prostate growth and inflammation. *Journal of Steroid Biochemistry & Molecular Biology* 2008; 108:254-260.

10. Chamie K, et al. Agent Orange exposure, Vietnam War veterans, and the risk of prostate cancer. *Cancer* 2008; 113:2464-2470.

11. Leitzmann MF, et al. Ejaculation frequency and subsequent risk of prostate cancer. *Journal of the American Medical Association* 2004; 291:1578-1686.

12. Holt SK, et al. Vasectomy and the risk of prostate cancer. *Journal of Urology* 2008; 180:2565-2567.

13. Huncharek M, et al. Smoking as a risk factor for prostate cancer: a meta-analysis of 24 prospective cohort studies. *American Journal of Public Health* 2010; 100:693-701.

14. Andriole GL, et al. Mortality results from a randomized prostate-cancer screening trial. *New England Journal of Medicine* 2009; 360:1310-1319.

15. Schröder FH, et al. Screening and prostate-cancer mortality in a randomized European study. *New England Journal of Medicine* 2009; 360:1320-1328.

16. Antonelliae JA, et al. Exercise and prostate cancer risk in a cohort of veterans undergoing prostate needle biopsy. *Journal of Urology* 2009; 182:2226-2231.

17. Lophatananon A; et al. Dietary fat and early-onset prostate cancer risk. *British Journal of Nutrition* 2010 [Epub ahead of print].

18. Aronson WJ, et al. Growth inhibitory effect of low fat diet on prostate cancer cells: results of a prospective, randomized dietary

intervention trial in men with prostate cancer. *Journal of Urology* 2010, 183:345-350.

19.   Kirsh VA, et al. Prospective study of fruit and vegetable intake and risk of prostate cancer. *Journal of the National Cancer Institute* 2007; 99:1200-1209.

20.   Lippman SM, et al. Effect of selenium and vitamin E on risk of prostate cancer and other cancers: the Selenium and Vitamin E cancer Prevention Trial (SELECT). *Journal of the American Medical Association* 2009; 301:39-51.

21.   Gaziano JM, et al. Vitamins E and C in the prevention of prostate and total cancer in men: the Physicians' Health Study II randomized controlled trial. *Journal of the American Medical Association* 2009; 301:52-62.

22.   Karppi J, et al. Serum lycopene and the risk of cancer: the Kuopio Ischaemic Heart Disease Risk Factor (KIHD) study. *Annals of Epidemiology* 2009; 19:512-518.

23.   Schwenke C, et al. Lycopene for advanced hormone refractory prostate cancer: a prospective, open phase II pilot study. *Journal of Urology* 2009; 181:1098-1103.

24.   Harper CE, et al. Genistein and resveratrol, alone and in combination, suppress prostate cancer in SV-40 tag rats. *Prostate* 2009; 69:1668-1682.

25.   Majid S, et al. Genistein reverse hypermethylation and induces active histone modifications in tumor suppressor gene B-Cell translocation gene 3 in prostate cancer. *Cancer* 2010; 116:66-76.

26.   Hwang YW, et al. Soy food consumption and risk of prostate cancer: a meta-analysis of observational studies. *Nutrition & Cancer* 2009; 61:598-606.

27.   Winkle K, et al. A phase II trial of a soy beverage for subjects without clinical disease with rising prostate-specific antigen after radical radiation for prostate cancer. *Nutrition & Cancer* 2010; 62:198-207.

28. Kurahashi N, et al. Plasma isoflavones and subsequent risk of prostate cancer in a nested case-control study: the Japan Public Health Center. *Journal of Clinical Oncology* 2008; 26:5923-5929.

29. Heald CL, et al. Phyto-oestrogens and risk of prostate cancer in Scottish men. *British Journal of Nutrition* 2007; 98:388-396.

30. Dalais FS, et al. Effects of a diet rich in phytoestrogens on prostate-specific antigen and sex hormones in men diagnosed with prostate cancer. *Urology* 2004; 64:510-515.

31. Shenouda NS, et al. Phytosterol Pygeum africanum regulates prostate cancer in vitro and in vivo. *Endocrine* 2007; 31:72-81.

32. Demark-Wahnefried W, et al. Flaxseed supplementation (not dietary fat restriction) reduces prostate cancer prostate cancer proliferation rates in men presurgery. *Cancer, Epidemiology, Biomarkers & Prevention* 2008; 17:3577-3587.

33. Cohen JH, et al. Fruit and vegetable intakes and prostate cancer risk. *Journal of the National Cancer Institute* 2000; 92: 61-68.

34. Kolonel LM, et al. Vegetables, fruits, legumes and prostate cancer: a multiethnic case-control study. *Cancer Epidemiology, Biomarkers & Prevention* 2000; 9: 795-804.

35. Ahn J, et al. Serum vitamin D concentration and prostate cancer risk: a nested case-control study. *Journal of the National Cancer Institute* 2008; 100:796-804.

36. Woo TC, et al. Pilot study: potential role of vitamin D (cholecalciferol) in patients with PSA relapse after definitive therapy. *Nutrition & Cancer* 2005; 51:32-36.

37. Kikuchi N, et al. No association between green tea and prostate cancer risk in Japanese men: the Ohsaki Cohort Study. *British Journal of Cancer* 2006; 95:371-373.

38. Kurahashi N, et al. Green tea consumption and prostate cancer risk in Japanese men: a prospective study. *American Journal of Epidemiology* 2008; 167:71-77.

39. McLarty J, et al. Tea polyphenols decrease serum levels of prostate-specific antigen, hepatocyte growth factor, and vascular endothelial growth factor in prostate cancer patients and inhibit production of hepatocyte growth factor and vascular endothelial growth factor in vitro. *Cancer Prevention Research* 2009; 2:673-682.

40. Rettig MB, et al. Pomegranate extract inhibits androgen-independent prostate cancer growth through a nuclear factor-kappa B-dependent mechanism. *Molecular Cancer Therapeutics* 2008; 7:2662-2671.

41. Pantuck AJ, et al. Phase II study of pomegranate juice for men with rising prostate-specific antigen following surgery of radiation for prostate cancer. *Clinical Cancer Research* 2006; 12:4018-4026.

42. Malik A & Mukhtar H. Prostate cancer prevention through pomegranate fruit. *Cell Cycle* 2006; 5: 371-373.

43. Rettig MB & Heber D. Pomegranate extract inhibits androgen-independent prostate cancer growth through a nuclear factor-kappa B-dependent mechanism. *Molecular Cancer Therapeutics* 2008; 7: 2662-2671.

44. Saleem M, et al. Lupeol inhibits proliferation of human prostate cancer cells by targeting beta-catenin signaling. *Carcinogenesis* 2009; 30:808-817.

45. Murtola TJ, et al. Prostate cancer and PSA among statin users in the Finnish prostate cancer screening trial. *International Journal of Cancer* 2010 [Epub ahead of print].

46. Thompson IM, et al. The influence of finasteride on the development of prostate cancer. *New England Journal of Medicine* 2003; 349:215-224.

47. Andriole GL, et al. Effect of dutasteride on the risk of prostate cancer. *New England Journal of Medicine* 2010, 362:1192-1202.

PART III

EPILOGUE

EPILOGUE

Contained within this single book is the cumulative wisdom and expertise of, literally, thousands of the world's brightest cancer scientists and clinicians, and the findings of hundreds of cutting-edge laboratory and clinical research studies in cancer prevention.

Devoid of fads, "too good to be true" advice, and breathless anecdotes, **A Cancer Prevention Guide for the Human Race** provides health-conscious readers with a comprehensive evidence-based approach to a healthy lifestyle that will help you to maximally reduce your risk of developing cancer. But all of the research studies in the world are of little use unless the knowledge and understanding that they provide are put to good and practical use. Therefore, I warmly urge you, Dear Readers, to apply the findings contained in this book to your daily lives, and to urge your loved ones to do the same.

May your lives be filled with love and hope, with good health, and with peace and contentment.

Robert A. Wascher, MD, FACS

www.doctorwascher.com

Irvine, California

June, 2010

CPSIA information can be obtained at www.ICGtesting.com
Printed in the USA
LVOW090858260812

295965LV00005B/121/P